A WEEK
to
CHANGE
YOUR
LIFE

A WEEK

to

CHANGE
YOUR
LIFE

HARNESS *the* POWER *of* YOUR BIRTHDAY
***and the* 7-DAY CYCLE THAT RULES YOUR HEALTH**

DR. OLIVIA AUDREY
with SARAH TOLAND

SIMON ELEMENT

New York London Toronto Sydney New Delhi

**SIMON
ELEMENT**

An Imprint of Simon & Schuster, Inc.
1230 Avenue of the Americas
New York, NY 10020

First Simon Element trade paperback edition February 2023

SIMON ELEMENT is a trademark of Simon & Schuster, Inc.

For information about special discounts for bulk purchases, please contact Simon & Schuster Special Sales at 1-866-506-1949 or business@simonandschuster.com.

The Simon & Schuster Speakers Bureau can bring authors to your live event. For more information or to book an event, contact the Simon & Schuster Speakers Bureau at 1-866-248-3049 or visit our website at www.simonspeakers.com.

Interior design by Jennifer Chung

Manufactured in the United States of America

10   9   8   7   6   5   4   3   2   1

Library of Congress Control Number: 2021946821

ISBN 978-1-9821-6911-4
ISBN 978-1-9821-6912-1 (pbk)
ISBN 978-1-9821-6913-8 (ebook)

Whether the universe is a concourse of atoms,
  or nature is a system, let this first be established,
    that I am a part of the whole which is governed by nature.

—*Marcus Aurelius*

CONTENTS

INTRODUCTION

No matter who you are or how you feel right now, nothing in your body is permanent—I promise. Any pain, illness, or upsetting symptoms you're experiencing are only temporary. Nothing in nature ever stays the same—your body, like everything else in the forests, oceans, deserts, and universe at large, is always changing, every second, every minute, every day, every week. With every change, you have an opportunity to feel better and heal. And that's what your body wants to do—to survive and thrive. Every organism, from the single-cell amoeba to the complicated trillions of cells that make up the human body, wants to survive. This means your body is designed to heal itself. All you have to do is let your body work its innate, universe-given magic that exists in every one of your cells.

Here's the truth: Your body knows what to do to be well. Every cell and organ inside you was created to resist disease, find balance, and maintain health and well-being. Your body is the smartest supercomputer humankind has ever known, constantly processing, using, and uploading data to create new neural pathways, cells, muscle adaptations, and emotional experiences that will help preserve and grow the expression of you in your environment. These are your body's bio-rhythms, the ancient wisdom that runs through each of us. All we have to do is stop, take a moment, and listen to these age-old rhythms. And while they may be quiet, the body's biorhythms are loud and clear once you know what to look for.

I started to learn about the body's biorhythms years ago, when I was just a little girl. I grew up in rural Maine in an off-the-grid communal living group where we grew our own food, carried our own water, and didn't have electricity—and where people used backwoods medicine, relying on plants, herbs, and intuitive healing to help make the body well. My mother, who gave birth to me home alone without even a midwife on hand, didn't take me to the doctor whenever I had an infection or took a nasty fall off a horse—instead, I was taught that my body would self-regulate and heal. You can imagine how surprised I was, then, when I started going to public school as a teen and saw all my friends popping Midol the minute they felt a cramp or seeing a doctor every time they had a cough or sore throat. The discrepancy between what had made me so healthy and what I saw in society sparked my interest in health care, and after graduating from high school, I enrolled in the University of North Carolina at Chapel Hill as a premed major.

Once at college, I was surprised that none of what I had experienced about the body's innate ability to heal was being taught—or even acknowledged. Instead, I got a deeper education on how conventional medicine treats illness: by using toxic drugs and invasive procedures to override the body's ability to self-regulate. In every fiber of my being, I knew this wasn't healing. To me, this wasn't preventative care—it was sick care. Conventional medicine only used and espoused techniques to treat people after they were seriously ill. I couldn't go forward with this kind of education in good conscience, and I dropped out of UNC.

My interest in medicine and healing didn't wane, though. After leaving UNC, I traveled around Central and South America, learning as much as I could about plant medicine and indigenous healing. Around the same time, my godmother suffered a heart attack. She was hospitalized and underwent a quadruple bypass—her first time ever being treated by Western medicine. As I learned about her rapid deterioration in conventional care, I knew I had to go back to my original mission to become a trained professional who could help the body heal on its own. I didn't want to go back to the school in the States, so I enrolled in Trinity College in Dublin, where I graduated with a degree in premed. Afterward, I went back to the US to study at the Trinity School of Natural Health in Indiana, where I became a board-certified naturopath. This means I have similar training as conventional doctors do, but I use natural medicine, not drugs and invasive interventions, to help treat disease or keep people feeling well before they ever get sick.

After I became a board-certified doctor, it was time for me to go home. I moved back to Maine, where I started treating friends, family, and other people I knew out of their homes. Many of my initial patients had difficult-to-treat conditions like hormone imbalances or stubborn weight gain. Some were very sick. As I started to help them overcome these seemingly incurable issues, usually without drugs or other conventional treatments, I earned a reputation as an out-of-the-box but highly effective healer. As demand for my kind of medicine increased, I opened two naturopathic clinics—one in Maine, the other in New Hampshire—and hired acupuncturists, massage therapists, Reiki healers, and similar alternative practitioners to help me use the power inherent in every patient's body to heal itself.

Both practices were immediately busy, primarily with patients who had serious illnesses like cancer and heart disease. These people wanted my help after conventional medicine had failed to treat their conditions or left them stuck feeling okay but never truly well. Many of them were receiving treatments that required frequent blood work, and as I drew more and more blood and reviewed their results over the years, I began to notice a really fascinating trend: Their inflammation levels seemed to spike one day each week, every week, after having been baseline only a few days prior, with no explainable change in disease progression. What's more, this inflammation spike occurred on the same day of the week for each patient, even though that day, whether it was a Monday or Friday, was wholly unique to them.

For months, I couldn't figure out why this spike was happening with such seven-day regularity. I pored over the research and spoke with many other doctors, but no one had noticed or recorded the phenomenon. The only thing that seemed to explain the occurrence was something called circaseptan rhythms, a theory that our bodies follow a seven-day clock just like it does a twenty-four-hour one, otherwise known as our circadian rhythms. Still, no one had used circaseptan rhythms to explain or even document why our bodies' inflammation levels would surge the same day of the week, week after week after week.

Over the next several years, I read everything about circaseptan rhythms I could find while conducting research on our apparent seven-day cycle and speaking with every credible doctor I knew. After a three-month study where I drew my patients' blood daily, I came to a startling conclusion: These circaseptan rhythms were what the body relied on to self-regulate and heal. The reason the body increases natural levels of inflammation every week is to trigger a comprehensive and consistent detoxification process. This detoxification process eliminates chronic or longer-lasting inflammation, which is the root cause of all disease.

This was genius on behalf of the body: Detoxification is what helps our bodies self-regulate in an internal and external environment where we're constantly bombarded by cellular waste, viruses, bacteria, stress, and other toxins that increase inflammation and eventually make us feel unwell. I knew if I could help people listen to their bodies and live their lives according to these seven-day rhythms like we already do our circadian rhythms by going to bed and getting up with the sun, I could help them lower inflammation and boost their bodies' ability to detoxify—two feats that would mitigate or even overturn almost any health ailment, big or small. This is how I developed the Protocol, a seven-day plan that aligns what you eat, how you exercise, and what you do on a daily basis to your body's seven-day rhythms in order to lower your inflammation levels and help your body better detoxify.

Over the past decade, I've used the same Protocol to treat hundreds of patients, including many A-list celebrities, pro athletes, and even royalty, and help them turn around their health and find new peace and vitality within. A patient with terminal cancer that chemotherapy and radiation hadn't been able to treat, for example, went into remission only several months after adopting the Protocol and after she had stopped all conventional treatment. A young man who had been prematurely bald at age twenty-eight saw his hair loss reversed in six months. An older man with distressingly high blood pressure and heart pain was suddenly symptom-free. All these results came when patients stopped trying to override their bodies' natural rhythms and started to listen to what their bodies wanted them to do, innately and intrinsically.

Listening to your body's biorhythms requires a different approach from anything else you've likely done in the past to improve your health, though. Tuning an ear to the quiet but powerful hum of your body's healing cycle may make you uncomfortable at first, but I believe that only when we get out of our comfort zones can we initiate the change that transforms our health, healing, and energy.

Over the years, I've learned to take the time to tune my own ear, listening to my patients and working with them to integrate their mind, body, and spirit together. We do this by talking about their home life, their daily environment, and the most difficult things they live with physically. Only after I dig into their physical reality do we begin to talk about their emotional and energetic being. I don't try to steer the conversation—I let them unfold. I find that when given the chance and space, people will offer up the most insightful clues to their own process. By doing this, I try to help every patient discover the highest expression of their own potential and peel back the layers of what has been there all along to help them feel holistically well.

If you currently feel frustrated, scared, or like you've hit a wall with your health, I want you to know that hope is much closer than it might feel. Your body already knows what to do—you just have to tap into its ancient wisdom. The Protocol realigns you with this wisdom and your body's natural forces, which are as powerful as the sun, moon, and tides. Like all celestial bodies, you are an integral and influential part of the universe, physically and spiritually. Physically, our bodies are made up of stardust—dust from stars that explode and fall into the earth's atmosphere.[1] Our cells share the same internal pattern as the most massive stars,[2] according to studies, and our brains contain as many cells as there are stars in the galaxy. This means you're literally a superstar who has all the power of the universe in every one of your cells. You breathe the same air on Earth and absorb the same material that every prophet, philosopher, poet, priest, physician, and healer before you has breathed and absorbed. You walk the planet just as Jesus, Buddha, Muhammad, and Mother Teresa did. You are just as powerful as they are, and you are every bit as much a healer.

But many of us have forgotten or lost touch with just how powerful we are. So many people feel disenfranchised by their bodies, believing that they're victims of their genetics, diseases, or both. Others feel like there's nothing they can do to change how they feel or look. This isn't low self-esteem; many of the same people feel empowered by their careers, families, or social lives, just not by their health.

That's what I want to change with this book—to empower you to take control of your own health by harnessing your body's ability to heal. And I can help you do that in one week's time, which is how long it takes to synchronize with your seven-day cycle, work with your body's rhythms, and start transforming your health, energy, and physical and emotional well-being. Since my first three-month study, I've conducted years of continued research and daily blood work on hundreds of patients to corroborate what I know to be occurring inside our bodies. I've made it my life's work to unravel the seven-day cycle and understand how our cells dance with our circaseptan rhythms and how we can learn to dance alongside them to be healthier, happier human beings.

Most books and online articles give facts and stats about the body, but not about *your* body. While interesting, these facts and stats aren't particularly revelatory or useful since everything about your health and well-being is unique to you. If healing was as simple as generic facts and stats, we'd all be able to do a quick Google search and cure whatever ails us. I'm not here for the generic. The Protocol in this book is all about you, your individual seven-day cycle, and how to sync with your unique rhythms that have been beating inside your body since the moment you were born.

To get on the path to empowerment, you first need one thing: an education in self. Knowledge is power, and this book is about putting the extraordinary powers of your body back into your control. As you learn about your seven-day cycle and how to live by the Protocol, you'll gain this knowledge for life and can choose to use it whenever and to whatever degree you want or need to.

I want you to believe that you have the power and the ability to heal what ails you. The first thing I do with any new patient is to debunk the myth that your body is static, confined by your genetics or your environment. Your body is anything but static—it's always changing and evolving, as I said at the beginning of this introduction. I know this not only because I'm a doctor but also because I'm an intuitive healer. This means that I approach illness from a more comprehensive place on a more esoteric level than most people do. I'm able to see where and how people are sick, in addition to using my training in medicine to diagnose them. Intuition has allowed me to see both sides of the fence in health care: I see science, I see intuition, and, oftentimes, I find my intuition to be more informative than my scientific understanding. And when it comes to understanding the body's seven-day cycle, my intuition has helped guide me more than a medical degree to see what happens inside us all.

As a naturopath and intuitive, I also like to keep things simple. While the Protocol is different than any other health plan, it's not complicated. You just want to align your body with what it has wanted to do since the day you were born. This makes the Protocol congenital, organic, and easy, and after a few weeks (or seven-day cycles), the plan will become second nature—because, after all, it *is* second nature, or what your body has always wanted to do.

In the post-pandemic era, understanding our bodies' power is more critical now than ever before. COVID-19 showed us many things, including how vulnerable we can become if we don't take care of our health and listen to our bodies. The outbreak forced many of us to take a hard look at how healthy we really are, and as a result, many have realized they're not as healthy as they thought they were. No one can afford to stay on autopilot about their health—we need to be more aware, more preventative, and more proactive.

Being proactive, however, doesn't just mean caring about your physical health: It also means caring for your emotional health. After all, you can't heal your body if you have too much trauma, whether that trauma is physical or emotional.

Trauma is anything that occurs to us, physically or emotionally, that can cause the body to be unwell. We all experience physical and emotional trauma, both major and minor, which the body can store for weeks, months, and even years. Just like trees record trauma in their trunks, developing different diameters of growth rings based on whether there was a draught, infestation, or fire, your body keeps score of your traumas internally, too, holding on to them until you release them. If you truly want to heal your body, it is critical for you to recognize and release your trauma, which means working to get over emotional pain as much as you do the physical stuff.

While emotional trauma may sound difficult to release, it's not when you do a little legwork. The Protocol helps heal emotional trauma by taking a 360-degree view—body, mind, and spirit—of how you live and feel on a day-to-day basis.

When you initiate this kind of total healing process and learn to live in rhythm with your body, mind, and spirit, everything in your life will flow more easily—every relationship, every career, every move you make, every activity you do. Suddenly, there's synergy.

Using this book, I want to help you find that synergy, tap into the power you have, and ultimately understand that you already have everything you need to live with radiant health. I see so many people suffer unnecessarily because they're holding themselves back. I'm here to tell you that you don't have to suffer anymore. You are powerful, you are the change, and you are the antidote.

Your body's ability to heal is greater than anyone has ever permitted you to believe. So let the healing begin.

THE SCIENCE OF SEVENS

CHAPTER 1

The first question I ask all my new patients is something no doctor has ever asked them before. I don't quiz them about their symptoms, prior medical history, or even the condition that made them make an appointment to see me in the first place. I don't need to know their blood type, cholesterol ratio, or results of their last blood work, MRI, or other diagnostic testing—I'll get there eventually, but not yet. I'm also not interested in knowing right off the bat what other doctors diagnosed them with or told them about their treatment options—I've been a naturopathic doctor and healer long enough to know that conventional doctors often get it wrong, drawing inaccurate conclusions or prescribing treatments that can do more harm than good.

Instead, the first thing I want to know from all my patients is the day of the week on which they were born. Not the month, day, or year but the actual day of the week—Monday, Tuesday, Wednesday, and so on—when they first entered this world as a living, breathing soul.

How is the day of the week of your birth even remotely related to your health and well-being? That is, in part, what this book is about. In short, knowing the day of the week on which you were born can help you finally—*finally!*—get in tune with your natural biorhythms and start working with your body rather than against it to heal, boost your energy, and get truly, organically, and holistically healthy.

You probably already know something about your body's *circadian* rhythms, or your twenty-four-hour biological clock that governs your sleep-wake cycles. If you've ever traveled to a different time zone, stayed up really late, or worked an overnight shift, you know how disrupting your circadian rhythms can affect your body, mind, and mood. If you get out of whack with your circadian rhythms, you'll feel tired, lethargic, and groggy. You may also have trouble focusing, coming up with new ideas, and thinking rationally. And if you're like most people, you'll also feel irritated, grouchy, uneasy, constantly hungry, and have low energy.

But disrupting your circadian rhythms doesn't just affect how you feel—your body also takes a big biological hit every time you interrupt this natural biorhythm. When you fall out of sync with your daily sleep-wake cycle, you'll increase your inflammation, interfere with your digestion, lower your immunity, and boost the kind of oxidative stress that can lead to weight gain, skin problems, premature aging, cognitive problems, and nearly every kind of chronic disease. In other words, when you don't live in accordance with your natural circadian rhythms, you're much more susceptible to not feeling or looking as good as you can, not to mention developing a serious disease.

Study after study corroborates what happens when people disrupt their circadian rhythms. Research has found that night owls, night-shift workers, and frequent time-zone travelers have an increased risk of weight gain, viral infections, heart disease, cancer, and other serious symptoms and illnesses. Studies have even found that people who work rotating night shifts for five years have an 11 percent higher risk of premature death than those who don't work overnight.[1]

What I'm telling you so far may not be necessarily new to you: Our circadian rhythms are well researched and well understood by conventional medicine. What's not so well-known, however, are the body's *circaseptan rhythms*, or the seven-day biological clock that dictates our inflammation levels, ability to heal, and energy flow in a similar way that our circadian rhythms do. While your primary-care doctor may have never heard of circaseptan rhythms (which is likely true of many other aspects of healing and holistic health), these seven-day rhythms are even more potent than your circadian clock. Circaseptan rhythms help control how well we feel, our day-to-day energy levels, whether we get sick, and how quickly or effectively we heal from illness, regardless of whether that illness is a major disease like cancer or a minor ailment like weight gain.

Because our seven-day cycle is so influential on our overall health, I've spent nearly my entire medical career studying it, developing a plan to help patients sync with their circaseptan rhythms (just like we do our circadian rhythms), and working with clients all over the world to overhaul their health using this plan. What I've learned after years of research is that the timing of our seven-day cycle isn't universal: Everyone's circaseptan clock starts on a different day of the week. And when your seven-day clock starts has everything to do with the day of the week on which you were born.

This makes total sense if you think about it: Your body basically pushed the "start button" on your seven-day cycle—and every other biorhythm in the body—

when you became a full-fledged human being and all your internal organs had to start working independently of your mother to live, breathe, and eat for yourself. In other words, every physiological process started the moment you were born, including the body's circaseptan rhythms. What this means is that if you were born on a Monday, your seven-day cycle started on a Monday and has repeated since then, week after week after week, in circaseptan regularity.

If you've never heard the term *circaseptan rhythms* before, you're not alone—most people haven't. But the concept has been studied by scientists at eminent organizations around the world, including the National Institutes of Health (NIH), for several decades. Research on circaseptan rhythms has also been published in the *Lancet*[2] and other prestigious medical journals.

Scientists at the NIH, for example, recognized that many illnesses, like high blood pressure, viral infections, and stroke, operate on a weekly clock, peaking once every seven days.[3] Since the concept of a seven-day week is also a socio-cultural construct, the researchers attributed these spikes to changes in behavior dictated by what we do during the week versus the weekend. For example, strokes and heart attacks are more likely to take place on a Monday, which researchers partially credit to the universal dread many feel returning to work and the fact that people often disrupt their circadian rhythms over the weekend by staying up later, drinking alcohol, et cetera.[4]

Other studies, however, have shown that there are biological reasons, not just social ones, to explain the existence of our seven-day rhythms. One study in the *Lancet*, for example, found that the manifestation of epilepsy in some patients operates on a seven-day clock, meaning they're more likely to have seizures once every week, on the same day of the week, over and over again.[5] Another study on pacemaker implants from the University of Minnesota found that many physiological processes occur on a seven-day cycle, including testosterone excretion and whether the body accepts or rejects a heart device.[6]

These studies are specific to certain conditions, but they show that scientists understand that some diseases and physiological processes have distinct circaseptan rhythms. What they don't understand, however, is exactly why certain physiological processes have seven-day cycles. But after years of research, I know why and have been able to document it in hundreds of patients.

Not only do some diseases and physiological processes have circaseptan rhythms but the body as a whole has a master circaseptan rhythm that dictates our levels of inflammation—the primary cause of illness and chronic disease—and how quickly we get rid of that inflammation, or when the body detoxifies. I call this our seven-day inflammation-detoxification cycle: Every week, the body increases inflammation, and every week it gets rid of that inflammation.

On the days of the week when the body is most inflamed, our energy is lower, and we're more prone to illness and injury. On the days of the week when the body detoxifies, we get rid of much of this inflammation, with the opportunity to clear even more harmful stuff from the body if we make smart decisions about what we do, eat, and drink. Following this inflammation spike and detoxification process—what I call the Cleanse—we're less inflamed, our energy is higher, we feel better, we're less bloated, we're cognitively sharper, we're emotionally more stable, we're better able to take on more difficult projects and do harder workouts in the gym, and we'll recover more quickly if we choose to travel.

Knowing your seven-day inflammation-detoxification cycle gives you a huge opportunity to make decisions every day that can help your body lower its inflammation and increase detoxification. Or you can do the opposite, stressing your body when it's most inflamed and slowing its ability to self-cleanse, self-regulate, and heal. Just like you can go to bed at night and wake up in the morning to sync with your circadian rhythms, you can also align your lifestyle choices with your circaseptan rhythms, making decisions about what you do and eat based on what's happening inside your body on a certain day of the week, according to your seven-day inflammation-detoxification cycle. And just as syncing with your circadian rhythms can help boost your energy, health, and overall well-being, aligning with your master circaseptan rhythm will help you overhaul your energy, lose weight, fight disease, improve the appearance of your skin, hair, and nails, clear your mind, boost your focus, and help prevent illness from happening in the first place. Remember, your master circaseptan rhythm is an even stronger clock than your circadian cycle.

What all this means is that learning about your seven-day inflammation-detoxification cycle gives you a huge opportunity: Basically, it empowers you to take control of your health and healing whenever you want or choose to live in accordance with your circaseptan rhythms. When you sync with your seven-day cycle, you're no longer a passive bystander in your own health and healing. Instead, you can wake up and make a choice every day to improve your energy, appearance, mental and emotional outlook, and overall health and well-being by making simple decisions about what you do and don't do. These choices can take a little work and, at times, may make you uncomfortable, but effecting real change in your body and your well-being requires getting out of your comfort zone. And that's what I want to help you see with this book: You can take control, and you do have the power to help your own body heal.

I know, I know: These are all big promises. And maybe they're promises you've been made before by other health books, plans, or protocols. But syncing with your body's seven-day cycle isn't like going on a new diet, trying a crazy exercise plan, doing a juice cleanse, or signing up for whatever other health or fitness fad is trending on Instagram. Instead, you're aligning with your body's ultimate internal clock—the same one that determines when and if you get sick and how well your body functions. It's not a fad: It's a way of life that can help you start to feel better and get healthier after just one week.

As a doctor, I've used the science of our master circaseptan rhythms and the plan I created around it to help treat hundreds of patients for a range of conditions, including major diseases like stage IV cancer, diabetes, and heart disease, in addition to less serious problems like hair loss, stubborn weight gain, brain fog, and menopausal symptoms. In some cases, my patients have been sick for years, even decades, and have already tried numerous types of treatments, none of which were effective until they started listing to their bodies' biorhythms.

I'm a naturopath—and for some, that may immediately bring to mind a vision of me swinging crystals over people's heads and chanting strange sounds. But that's not how I practice. And my patients aren't those you might think would necessarily see a naturopath. I help treat lots of everyday people, of course, but I've also worked with dozens of A-list celebrities. These famous people, many of whom have access to some of the best doctors in the world, choose to work with me because I can help them in ways no other physician can, steering them to make simple choices about their daily actions that finally get them in sync with their bodies' organic rhythms, transforming their everyday health, healing, and energy levels.

Before I go into more detail about our seven-day inflammation-detoxification cycle and how you can sync with yours to be healthier and happier, I think it's really important to understand more of the science behind circaseptan rhythms, why and how the body functions on a seven-day cycle, and what I call the science of sevens, which is the remarkable presence of sevens in nature, religion, culture, the human body, and time eternal.

Why the *When* Matters
More Than the *How* or *How Much*

While circaseptan rhythms aren't necessarily mainstream medical knowledge, the field of chronomedicine, or chronotherapy, has been around for decades—and is gaining more and more attention as doctors realize how powerful the practice can be. Chronomedicine uses the body's biological rhythms—the internal time clocks that we all have—to optimize medical treatment, drug delivery, and overall health and well-being. The practice has been around since the 1970s, when researchers first discovered that mice infected with cancer could be treated more effectively by taking drugs at different points throughout the day, based on the biological rhythms inside the rodents.[7]

Since the '70s, research on chronomedicine has exploded, as scientists have discovered that the timing of a patient's treatment can matter as much as the treatment itself. A recent study published in the *Lancet*, for example, found that patients who undergo heart surgery in the afternoon suffer fewer complications than those who have the same procedure in the morning because levels of certain heart-protective proteins increase as the day goes on.[8] On the other hand, scientists at Washington University found that patients who take cancer medication in the morning respond better than those who take the same drugs at night.[9] Some cancer patients for whom traditional treatment hasn't worked have gone into remission simply by switching the timing of their medication, according to the scientific journal *Nature*.[10]

You don't need to be scheduled for heart surgery or undergoing cancer treatment to benefit from the findings on chronotherapy. Research on chronomedicine has also shown that taking aspirin before bed instead of in the morning can cut the risk of heart attack and stroke in half.[11] Similarly, doctors have found that taking statin medications at night is more effective, since the body typically produces cholesterol during the overnight hours.[12] Taking too much acetaminophen (or the brand name, Tylenol) in the morning can be toxic to the liver, while the same dose at night doesn't appear to have as detrimental an effect.[13]

There are dozens of other examples of how timing affects disease treatment, but what chronomedicine shows us is that the biological rhythms in our bodies matter hugely to our overall health. According to Robert Dallmann, who studies the body's internal molecular-clock biology at the Warwick Medical School in England, "We have clocks in our bodies that control most physiological processes. They determine when we are active, when we rest, and how we metabolize drugs."[14]

Plenty of scientists are still eager to investigate chronomedicine and learn more about our biological rhythms and how we can leverage them to better treat disease and improve our overall health. In 2017, for example, the Nobel Prize in Physiology or Medicine was awarded to three American researchers who discovered a gene that increases protein production at different times over a twenty-four-hour period.[15] While most of us know that the body's sleep-wake cycle follows a circadian rhythm, these scientists are proving that other significant physiological functions also operate on very specific time clocks. And we're just skimming the tip of the iceberg.

Much of the research on chronomedicine is nascent, innovative, and continually evolving. Just because a certain biological rhythm hasn't been widely researched or even documented yet by the world's leading scientists doesn't mean it doesn't exist. Throughout this book, I would encourage you to trust in the fact that your body, just like the sun, moon, ocean, and almost everything around us in nature, has a unique set of rhythms, some of which we know about and others that remain a mystery. Either way, looking inward and learning to listen to your own internal rhythms, just like paying attention to when the sun rises and sets, can make all the difference to your overall energy, health, and well-being.

This Is the Rhythm of Your Life

So far, we've talked a lot about biological rhythms. But what exactly are our biological rhythms, which, for the purpose of this book, we'll also refer to as our bodies' internal clocks? Let's take a look.

The body has a number of different biological rhythms or clocks. Some, like our sleep-wake cycle, run on a circadian (daily) cycle while others, like body temperature, are circasemidian, meaning they peak twice (semidaily) over the course of a twenty-four-hour period. Some biological rhythms, like heart rate and appetite, happen so frequently in the body that they're ultradian, meaning they occur multiple times per day, while others, like breeding, seasonal weight gain, and hibernation in some animals, are considered to be infradian, with cycles lasting much longer than a twenty-four-hour period.

Of all the body's internal clocks, the most influential are our circaseptan rhythms, which mean they occur inside our bodies on a seven-day cycle.

Perhaps you're wondering why the body would operate on a seven-day cycle. After all, isn't the seven-day week a man-made concept and thereby arbitrary? Yes and no. While the seven-day week is certainly a sociocultural construct, there's a reason the ancient Babylonians, who created the idea of a seven-day week, chose the number seven: They based it on the cycle of the moon.[16] A single phase of the moon lasts approximately seven days, or one full week. There are four phases of the moon, which occur over the course of twenty-eight days—what we perceive to be a calendar month. This means that every seven-day week marks a new lunar phase, and every month marks a full lunar cycle.

While the moon certainly affects our physical and mental health—studies show lunar cycles can influence our sleep, mood, and some other parameters of overall health and well-being[17]—the body's circaseptan rhythms exceed the presence of seven-day lunar phases. In short, we don't necessarily know why the body keeps circaseptan rhythms any more than we know why we have circadian rhythms. But both exist in our bodies and seem to play a fascinating role in our ability to heal.

The father of medicine, Greek physician Hippocrates, recognized the importance of our seven-day cycle thousands of years ago when he determined that disease occurs on seven-day schedules, lasting seven, fourteen, or twenty-one days and, whenever fatal, taking its victims on the seventh day after the onset of illness.[18]

Hippocrates aside, how could the most influential rhythm in the body be one that you've never heard of? There are many things in science and medicine that most people, even doctors, either don't know about or don't pay attention to, despite there being a direct correlation between the information and good health. For example, think about good nutrition: When was the last time you detailed for your doctor what you were eating on a daily basis or you received a prescription for more green veggies and less sugar? Circaseptan rhythms are similar: Just because you haven't chatted with your doctor about your seven-day cycle doesn't mean it's not imperative to your overall health.

Dozens of critical biological processes within the body have circaseptan rhythms. One profound example is cell mitosis—the process by which a cell divides into two daughter cells. Every seven days, many cells, including white and red blood cells, divide to create new cells. The epithelial cells that line our intestine also regenerate every five to seven days,[19] helping to refurbish our microbiome—the trillions of microorganisms that live inside our guts and influence our health, mood, and overall well-being. Because cell mitosis occurs on a seven-day cycle, we have the ability to influence whether we create healthy or unhealthy new cells every week, as the body regenerates. We'll delve into this in greater detail throughout the book.

The first seven days after conception, a fertilized egg divides multiple times to become an embryo, eventually implanting around the seven-day mark into the uterus.[20] That makes these first seven days critical to the viability of an embryo—it's the embryo's time to make it or break it, when it multiplies from one cell to several hundred. Half of all embryos don't successfully implant, so if an embryo makes it past the one-week mark, it's got a fighting chance of survival.[21] (Note that the body's seven-day inflammation-detoxification cycle doesn't start in the womb since much of a fetus's organ, immune, and overall function is dependent on the mother.)

A woman's menstrual cycle also follows a seven-day cycle—four weekly cycles, to be exact, culminating in menstruation every twenty-eight days. During the first week of a woman's cycle, her estrogen increases, boosting mood and energy.[22] During the second week, estrogen continues to climb while her testosterone also increases, ratcheting up her energy and confidence while suppressing appetite.[23] At the fourteen-day mark, a woman ovulates before starting the third week of her cycle, when the hormone progesterone starts to increase, making her more tired, sensitive, and hungry.[24] During the last week of her cycle, both estrogen and progesterone plummet, causing a woman to bleed while driving up feelings of anxiety, sadness, irritability, and appetite.[25]

Menstruation and cell mitosis aren't the only biological processes that follow circaseptan rhythms—there are dozens more, perhaps most notably in the immune system. For example, the body's two primary immune cells, T cells and B cells, peak and trough on a weekly basis, making us more or less susceptible to illness at different times throughout the week.[26] Animal studies have also shown that it takes about seven days for blood to develop antibodies after inoculation, although researchers are not sure why.[27]

Perhaps even more interestingly, the immune systems of people who suffer from cancer also appear to follow a six- to seven-day cycle, with inflammation and disease activity increasing and decreasing over the course of one week, according to one study.[28] Researchers made this discovery after tracking something called C-reactive protein (CRP)—a primary marker of inflammation in the blood that I've also tracked in my patients—in twenty-one cancer patients, noticing it peaked and troughed over the course of seven days. While they say more research is needed, scientists involved in the study believe that these results suggest cancer therapies could be individualized to a patient's oscillating CRP, either at peak or trough times, to be more effective.[29] The discovery of a seven-day immune cycle specific to cancer patients has been heralded by some as "the biggest breakthrough in modern cancer medicine,"[30] as researchers continue to investigate how to best time chemotherapy and other treatments to a patient's individual immune cycle.

Circaseptan rhythms also play a role in how the immune system responds to one of the most invasive medical procedures possible: organ transplantation. After a patient receives a new organ, he or she is required to stay in the hospital at least one full week—the proven length of time it takes to see whether the body either accepts or rejects the new organ.[31] Seven days after a transplant operation—and every seven days thereafter—patients receive immunosuppressive drugs.[32] While more research is needed, researchers speculate that the function of our immune cells as well as when the body's tissue regenerates both occur in seven-day cycles.[33]

The largest study on circaseptan rhythms to date, conducted on more than 1,100 patients, found that epilepsy can follow a seven-day cycle, with 23 percent of those in the study more prone to having seizures on one particular day of the week.[34] Since most patients had circadian (daily) seizure cycles in the study, researchers called the discovery of a precise seven-day seizure cycle in over one-fifth of the patient pool "staggering."[35] They added that a patient's high-seizure day was specific to him or her, which they hoped to use to better tailor a person's individual medication timing and other treatment.[36] At the same time, scientists involved in the study said they didn't know what causes seizure cycles to occur with daily or weekly regularity.

Other illnesses follow a seven-day cycle, too, including many viral and bacterial infections. If you get sick with the common cold, malaria, pneumonia, or COVID-19, for example, you'll likely either recover or spiral downward at the seven-day mark, according to science. In the instance of the coronavirus, the phenomenon is so acute that doctors now call it the "seven-day COVID-19 crash"—the one-week point at which hospitalized patients quickly deteriorate after showing prior signs of stability.[37] Because of the circaseptan nature of these illnesses, many treatments, including antibiotic drugs for infections, are typically prescribed for seven-day cycles, whether that's one week, two weeks, or even three weeks.

What happens at seven days to produce this make-or-break moment in so many viral and bacterial illnesses? The answer has to do with cytokines, proteins inside the body that tell immune cells what to do. Cytokines are a natural part of the immune system's response to any illness or foreign invader, but sometimes our immune system goes too far and produces a "cytokine storm," releasing too many cytokines into the blood, which begin to attack our own cells. But this process doesn't happen overnight; instead, cytokine storms generally take seven days to develop after the first signs of illness.

In addition to cell mitosis and our immune response to illness and surgery, our bodies have other profound circaseptan rhythms. We ramp up production of many endogenous chemicals like our sex hormones on a weekly basis. With women, fluctuations of estrogen and progesterone occur over four seven-day periods, making up their twenty-eight-day menstrual cycles. Men's testosterone levels also peak every seven days, sometimes by as much as an incredible 45 percent.[38]

While there's still a lot more research we can and should do on our circaseptan rhythms, what science has already shown us is that many biological processes and illnesses operate on a seven-day schedule. We'll go into much greater detail about how we can use this knowledge to help prevent or fight illness and boost our overall health, but first I want to look at the number seven and its significance in nature, religion, culture, and the universe at large.

While the number seven has more mysticism than science, I've found that helping people understand how powerful the number seven is inside the human body and brain and throughout society and history helps them make better sense of their own seven-day cycle. For me and millions of others, seven is a really romantic number and can help empower you to embark on the journey to line up with your own seven-day cycle. When you realize the mystical importance of seven, you can see yourself as part of something bigger. Even if you don't entirely understand the science we just covered, you can understand the symbolism of seven and that you're part of a divine matrix, one you can lean into by living in sync with your master circaseptan rhythm.

The Science of Sevens in the Brain

Human beings love the number seven, mentally, emotionally, and spiritually. It's our favorite number, our lucky number, and the number we most often see or remember when given or shown a variety of options.

One of the best-known principles in psychology is the "magical number seven," which posits that our short-term memory can only hold seven items at a time.[39] Penned by American psychologist George Miller in the 1950s, "The Magical Number Seven, Plus or Minus Two" states that our brains can store seven units of information, plus or minus two. This is why phone numbers are seven digits long (not including area codes)[40] and why if you're shown a collection of items on an empty table, you'll likely be able to remember only a maximum of seven.[41]

Since Miller published his classic essay on the magical number seven, researchers have come up with a scientific reason why our short-term memory likes the number seven so much. Our brain cells, or neurons, produce the best information when they have seven dendrites, or branches, that receive stimulation.[42]

In part for this reason, our minds are also attracted to the number seven when we scan for information and group details. If you look at popular book titles, movies, and articles written in list format, otherwise known as listicles, you'll find most include seven points. For example, *The 7 Habits of Highly Effective People* by Stephen Covey is one of the world's best-selling books, with more than forty million copies sold in fifty languages since it was first published in 1989.[43]

Scan other bestseller lists and you'll also find *The Seven Spiritual Laws of Success* by Deepak Chopra, *Seven Pillars of Wisdom* by T. E. Lawrence, *The Seven Principles for Making Marriage Work* by John M. Gottman and Nan Silver, and *Seven Myths of the Spanish Conquest* by Matthew Restall—the list goes on. Similarly, Hollywood has discovered that the number seven has emotional appeal when placed in movie titles, with *The Seven Year Itch*, *Seven Years in Tibet*, *Seven Samurai*, *The Magnificent Seven*, *Seven Minutes in Heaven*, the Up series of films (*Seven Up!*, *7 Plus Seven*, *21 Up*, etc.), and dozens more, all blockbuster hits.

We as human beings also just like the number seven, plain and simple. When British mathematician Alex Bellos asked forty-four thousand people around the world to pick their favorite number, seven was the top choice.[44] Bellos hypothesized that people like the number seven because it feels magical and unique. He also pointed out it's the only number within the grouping one through ten that can't be multiplied or divided to achieve a result within the grouping (one, two, three, four, and five can be doubled; six, eight, and ten can be halved; and nine divides by three).[45]

Culturally, humans also think the number seven is lucky. You've likely heard the phrase "lucky number seven." In Las Vegas, you'll hit the jackpot on a slot machine with the triple-seven line, while seven is the number to bet on the pass line in craps. Opposite sides of a die add up to the number seven, which is also the number most likely to occur when you roll two standard six-sided dice.

Seven is also considered a lucky number in China, Japan, and many other cultures around the world. The number is represented in some of these countries' ancient healing practices, too. In traditional Chinese medicine, for example, women follow a seven-year cycle of development, with specific physiological functions occurring at age seven, fourteen, twenty-one, twenty-eight, and so on.[46] Reiki, or the Japanese practice of energy healing, focuses on aligning the seven chakras, or energy centers, in the body. In the ancient Indian practice of Ayurveda, there are seven basic constitutions (pitta, kapha, vata, vata-pitta, vata-kapha, pitta-kapha, and vata-pitta-kapha).[47]

The Science of Sevens in Nature, Religion, Culture, and History

In nature, the science of sevens is everywhere. As you now know, each phase of the moon lasts approximately seven days, which also pulls the ocean into circaseptan rhythms, as maximum high tide occurs seven days after the neap tide, when water levels are at their lowest. There are also seven continents, corresponding to the seven major tectonic plates in Earth's continental crust, and seven seas. There are seven colors of the rainbow, as water droplets break white sunlight into seven colors of the spectrum, and seven different types of electromagnetic waves, including radio waves, microwaves, infrared, optical, ultraviolet, X-rays, and gamma rays.

In chemistry, a pH value of seven is the neutral marker between acidity and alkalinity. Only seven energy levels are needed to contain all the electrons in an atom, with seven rows in the periodic table to reflect the different categorization. There are seven pitches in a diatonic scale—a major scale that makes up the foundation of Western music—with five whole tones and two semitones (this five-to-two ratio will reappear throughout this book, too).

We see the number seven in living creatures, too. Most notably, there are seven life processes: movement, respiration, sensitivity, growth, reproduction, excretion, and nutrition. All mammals, except for sloths and manatees, have seven cervical vertebrae,[48] while the common ladybug that many of us grew up admiring has seven spots. Human skin is made up of seven different layers to protect our muscles, bones, and internal organs, while there are seven external holes in the human head: two eyes, two nostrils, two ears, and one mouth.

Outside of nature, the number seven is hugely significant in religion and culture. Perhaps the best-known example is the creation narrative in Christianity and Judaism, which holds that God created the heavens and the earth in six days, taking the seventh day to rest. In various faiths, we also see seven deadly sins, seven virtues, seven gifts of the Holy Spirit, seven joys of the Virgin Mary, seven days of the feast of Passover, and seven pairs of each animal brought onto the ark by Noah.

In classical antiquity, there are seven wonders of the ancient world, seven sages of Greece, seven hills of Rome, seven heroes against Thebes, and seven classical planets—the number of moving astronomical objects we can see with the naked eye from Earth. In Islam, there are seven levels of heaven and hell, while in Hinduism, there are seven chakras, seven seas in the world, seven worlds in the universe, and seven *rishis*, or gurus. In Buddhism, there are also seven factors of awakening, and Buddha is said to have taken seven steps at the time of his birth.

These systems of belief around seven are not accidental: They have survived for thousands of years for a reason. The number seven is an organic and mythical number for the human race, part of our spirituality as much as it is our biology.

Culturally, we see the number seven appear in almost every epoch of time and area of the world. In Western literature alone, the number holds mythical import. The Greek poet Homer couldn't get away from seven in his classical works: The hero Odysseus, for example, spends seven years in captivity, while other action in the *Odyssey* continues for six days before climaxing on the seventh day in some critical event. Shakespeare wrote about the seven ages of man, the Brothers Grimm about the seven dwarfs in *Snow White*, and T. A. Barron about the seven songs of Merlin in his classic trilogy the Lost Years of Merlin. Magical seven-league boots are used throughout fairy tales, allowing characters to take seven leagues per step and outpace their villains or simply the constraints of the human stride.

According to Western folklore, you'll incur seven years' bad luck if you break a mirror. Other idioms with the number seven abound, including the seven-year itch, or the time it takes for a relationship to run its course, and the seven-day wonder, which is when someone or something creates curiosity or fame for only a short period of time. More recently, the kissing game "seven minutes in heaven" has become the title of movies and songs, while there are seven games in most playoff series in Major League Baseball, the National Basketball Association, and the National Hockey League.

We can look to nearly every culture in Asia, Africa, and South America and find the significance of seven there, throughout time and various nationalities. What the examples prove is not that seven is a revolutionary number. It's not. In fact, it's just the opposite: It is so fundamental to our lives that we don't even realize it's there. What's important to keep in mind is that seven has meaning. And as we'll see in the next chapter, that meaning can change your life.

Learning what medical science has already shown us about the body's circaseptan rhythms, as well as the meaning of the number seven in the world at large, can help you better grasp what I'm about to share in the next few chapters. While it's not documented by any study or major clinical organization—this is my discovery as a spiritual healer after conducting blood work on hundreds of patients—our bodies follow a precise seven-day cycle of inflammation and detoxification that's unique to each of us, based on the day of the week on which we were born.

If you can shift your habits to align with your own seven-day cycle, you can reap the benefits that the theory of chronomedicine suggests, turning any disease around on a dime while improving your energy and preventing your body from getting sick in the first place. This means incredible health and healing are in your hands. All you have to do is learn how to line up with your powerful seven-day cycle that has been ebbing and flowing inside you since the moment you were born.

UNDERSTANDING
YOUR SEVEN-DAY CYCLE

CHAPTER 2

I t was a Monday. And I knew what Mondays meant for Katie.*

Whenever the thirty-seven-year-old came to see me on a Monday at my medical office in New Hampshire, she would always be tired, achy, and bloated. I knew I'd be getting the irritable and scatterbrained Katie, not the calmer, more centered mother of two she told me she was most other days of the week. On Mondays, Katie would say she didn't feel well, which was understandable since she had stage IV lymphoma. But it was always on a Monday when she *really* didn't feel well.

At the time, I was operating two naturopathic medical clinics—one in New Hampshire and the other in Maine. At both clinics, I specialized in using progressive, nonconventional remedies to help treat all kinds of illnesses. The fact that I was willing to think and treat outside the box attracted a lot of people for whom Western medicine had already failed. Like Katie, many of my patients had serious diseases and had been given only years or even months to live. They had explored nearly every avenue Western medicine could offer yet were not seeing the results that they wanted. These patients were at the end of their rope and were willing to try anything for a chance at survival.

Katie was no different. She had done chemotherapy, radiation, and immunotherapy, but these conventional treatments—the standard for cancer care in Western medicine—hadn't worked. When she came to me, I did something none of her other doctors had done before: I took a hard look at her diet and discussed with her what toxins she unknowingly might be exposing herself to every day. We also talked about how her emotional health could be impacting her physical health. When it came to her diet, I asked her to cut out dairy[1] and meat.[2] I also told her to stop using antiperspirant and conventional beauty products, which are full of known carcinogens. Emotionally, she wasn't in a good place, with a nega-

---

tive outlook on her job and, more so, her relationship with her mother. I told her we needed to work to resolve this negativity or it would continue to eat her up inside and prevent her from feeling fully well.

I also started drawing Katie's blood every week, which we did on a Monday because it was the easiest day of the week for her to get to my office—why I knew she was often irritable and sick on Mondays. Katie's blood results also corroborated what she was feeling: Inevitably, she'd have high levels of C-reactive protein—the body's primary indicator of inflammation—and other signs that her cancer wasn't improving.

It was only by happenstance that I discovered that these results, along with the Monday Katie I came to know, were only giving me part of the story.

How I Discovered the Seven-Day Cycle

One Monday, several months into our work together, Katie's son had a soccer game that she wanted to attend, so she switched our weekly appointment and blood draw to Wednesday. When she came to see me then, I noticed immediately that she looked and sounded better. She had more energy and appeared to be less bloated and puffy. She was more pleasant, focused, and even happier. When I asked her how she felt, she told me she wasn't as tired or achy as she had been earlier in the week.

Where I noticed the biggest difference, though, was in Katie's blood results. When we drew her blood that Wednesday, I couldn't believe what I saw: Her levels of C-reactive protein and other inflammatory markers were significantly lower. All of a sudden, her cancer seemed to be showing incredible signs of improvement.

The following Monday, Katie's son had another soccer game, so she came to see me on a Wednesday again. Just like the week before, the woman who showed up in my office midweek was a distinctly different person than the one who had typically come to see me earlier in the week. Similar to the previous Wednesday, Katie had more pep in her step, her face appeared less puffy, and she seemed calmer and happier. More impressively, her blood results showed much less inflammation, suggesting that her cancer was turning a corner.

Katie came to see me one more Wednesday, showing the same improvements in her appearance, demeanor, and inflammatory markers, before returning to her regular Monday schedule. Suddenly, the old Katie was back. She was tired, achy, irritable, and bloated. She told me she didn't feel well, and worse still, her blood results showed the same high levels of inflammation that they had three weeks ago. What was going on?

I began to realize that I was seeing a pattern: Whenever I drew Katie's blood on a Monday, her inflammation levels were sky-high. Monday was always the day when she didn't feel, look, sound, or act as well as she did during the other days of the week.

At first, I assumed something was happening on the weekends that was stressing Katie out or otherwise causing her to come into my office on Monday significantly sicker than the other days of the week. But over time, I began to see a similar pattern in some of my other patients: Almost all of them had days of week when they didn't respond as well to treatment, struggled during patient analysis, and had consistently poor lab results. It wasn't the same day of the week for each patient—for example, some were always cranky, sick, and tired on Mondays like Katie, while others were that way on a Tuesday, Wednesday, Thursday, or Friday. No matter which day was the bad day, it was the same day of the week for the same person, week after week after week. Their blood work would always be off the day when they were the crankiest and most tired, with significantly higher levels of inflammation than the rest of the week.

I began to wonder: What was going on inside these patients that was causing their inflammation, mood, and overall well-being to fall off the cliff the same day of the week, every week? I had to find out and decided to conduct my own research in order to do so. I asked twenty-five patients if they'd be amenable to having their blood drawn every single day of the week for three months' time so that I could track exactly what was happening on a weekly basis with their inflammation levels. To my delight, all twenty-five agreed, and with the help of some of the other practitioners in both my Maine and New Hampshire offices, we started drawing their blood on a daily basis.

After three months, the pattern couldn't have been clearer: All twenty-five patients had one day of the week when their inflammatory markers spiked considerably, showing higher levels of C-reactive protein, certain hormones, uric acid, and ketones (these last two substances are produced by the body as cellular waste and can indicate inflammation when present in excess). It wasn't the same day of the week for each patient, but it was the same day of the week for the same patient, week after week after week.

For example, one female patient's levels of uric acid would be 2.8 mg/dL on a Monday (within normal range for a woman) but 6.5 mg/dL on a Thursday (out of normal range), with that spike happening every Thursday for three months.

Yet for another female patient, uric acid spiked on a Sunday, while another patient's uric acid peaked on a Tuesday.

For many of my patients, the inflammation spike they experienced one day of the week was significant—up to 45 percent higher than what we established was their baseline the rest of the week. To put this percentage into perspective, a 45 percent spike in inflammation over baseline is what you might see if someone had just endured the physical trauma of a car accident or invasive surgery. But unlike in the instance of these events, the once-weekly spike in inflammation I saw in my patients was never sustained for more than one day: Blood work showed that their markers would plummet the next day and return to baseline over the course of the next several days before starting to build again by the end of the week. It was like a consistent and well-orchestrated symphony, happening over and over again, culminating in a one-day crescendo that dominated the musical piece.

After recognizing there was always an inflammation surge and subsequent drop, I realized what else had to be happening in my patients around the same time their inflammation was peaking: Their bodies had to be going through an intense detoxification process to get rid of all that inflammation and waste. It was the only way their blood results would be able to return to relative normal the following day.

But why was this happening? What was the reason behind this one-day inflammation surge and subsequent detoxification? As soon as I figured out the rhythm in my patients, these questions began to plague me night and day. It was like a Rubik's Cube I couldn't solve—I knew there had to be a biological reason behind the pattern; I just couldn't figure it out. I started racking my brain for possibilities, often waking up in the middle of the night with another idea or inspiration. It was similar to when I worked as a waitress in college and would wake up at five in the morning wondering if I ever brought table eight their ketchup. Now I was waking up at five in the morning wondering whether the timing of a patient's inflammation surge was related to a genetic variant, their mother's ethnicity, or another obscure factor.

At the same time, I began poring through all the medical literature I could find, trying to see if there was anything in any existing research on the existence of a seven-day cycle and why a patient's inflammation might spike one day of the week. What I discovered was *The Biology of Belief* by stem cell biologist Bruce Lipton, who talked about our circaseptan rhythms—a term I had never heard before at the time—and how the body behaved in accordance with the rhythms of the body. In the book, Lipton detailed animal studies he had done where altering the sleep cycles of mice by even an hour or two per night over the course of seven days effectively changed the outcome of cancer, causing tumor growth to stop altogether in one week.

I was blown away: The presence of circaseptan rhythms in the body was 100 percent the reason why people's blood was surging one day of the week, every week. Why didn't everyone know this? Why wasn't this something every doctor who had to review blood results talked about regularly?

Still, the awareness of circaseptan rhythms among some parts of the scientific community didn't explain why we all had a different day of the week when our inflammatory markers spiked. After all, we were all human beings—why didn't our inflammation surge happen on the same day of the week for all of us? I needed to do more research.

At the time, my experiment with my patients had been purely biological: I was only drawing blood and analyzing their physiological markers. Now I began to wonder if there was also an emotional aspect that I was overlooking. After all, our emotions significantly affect our physical health. Even traditional Western medicine acknowledges that anxiety and depression can increase the risk of serious illness,[3] while people who suffer traumas in early childhood, like the death of a parent, are at a far greater risk of getting sick as adults.[4]

While continuing to draw their blood, I also began interviewing patients about what their childhood was like, what traumas they could recall, and the last time they remember feeling really well. I asked them for their definition of love, wellness, happiness, and balance, along with what it meant to feel good—I wanted to get a scope of what their experience had been with their own well-being so far and how they thought their bodies felt in everyday life. We didn't talk about hopes and dreams—I wanted to uncover how they got to where they were, with the illnesses or ailments they had, so we focused on their fears and what might be holding them back from feeling good. I'm not a psychologist or psychiatrist, and I wasn't trying to psychoanalyze them, but I wanted to see if there could be an emotional connection to why each patient had his or her own unique seven-day cycle.

More than a month into my interviews, I was floored: Most of my patients had one day of the week when most of their life's traumas had occurred—and it was the same day of the week when their inflammation peaked. For example, one patient told me about losing a pregnancy on the day of the week when her inflammatory markers were the highest. Katie's grandmother, who helped her deal with the unhappy relationship she had with her mother, died on a Monday, the same day of the week when Katie's inflammation surged. Another patient told me about finding out on the day her inflammation levels were highest that her husband had cheated on her. The impact that these events had had on my patients made sense from a medical perspective, too: The body was more prone to illness or trauma, whether physical or emotional, when inflammation was highest. That's not to say that the events themselves were created by the patients' levels of inflammation, but the impact they made was heightened. But this still didn't account for why we had this seven-day inflammation-detoxification cycle in the first place and why each of our cycles took place on different days.

One warm September day near the end of my three-month experiment, I was sitting in the backyard of my home in Maine, enjoying the nature around me and being present in the moment. For this reason, I wasn't thinking about my research at the time but gazing instead at the rolling hills beyond the edge of my backyard, which was lined by maple ash and birch trees. I began to think about how the trees were so singularly beautiful yet so hardy to be able to withstand the harsh Maine winters. How did they do it? I thought about how trees record their trauma in growth rings deep beneath their bark—every year, trees form a new ring in their trunk, which reflects their health and whether they receive enough water and sunlight. I started to wonder where the human body would keep score if it could.

Then it hit me like a lightning bolt: Our seven-day cycle is the body's way of keeping score, our equivalent of growth rings. We record our growth every week just like a tree records its growth each year. What I was seeing in all my patients wasn't just a fluke—this was real, replicated by science and nature. We are replications of an older, more innate, and intricate scope of biology. The trees and animals have it right: Follow the nuances and rhythms of nature. It seems to be only humans who haven't fully realized the message in this ancient wisdom.

I went back to my office and pulled out all my patient notes, scouring the dates on their charts to try to identify a pattern that would connect their seven-day cycles with their general life span. I started googling calendars for each of my patients' birthdays, and suddenly, the dates started to line up like the matrix on a winning Powerball ticket: With every patient, the day of the week that their inflammation surged was the same day of the week on which they were born. Their birth was the trauma that launched their master circaseptan rhythm, and since that day, their bodies had been keeping score by recording the trauma of birth over and over again, spiking inflammation just like trees record trauma in their growth rings every year.

With this discovery in mind, I started reaching out to epidemiologists at the CDC who had studied circaseptan rhythms in viruses, doctors who understood that the body adheres to a seven-day schedule when it accepts or rejects an organ transplant, and authors who had published scientific papers on circaseptan rhythms. I figured someone had to be familiar with this phenomenon I had just discovered.

While I found crumbs in some published research—for example, that circaseptan rhythms could be responsible for the individual seven-day cycles of immune response in cancer and epileptic patients—no study I read or doctor I spoke with could corroborate the idea that we had a seven-day inflammation-detoxification cycle that was tied to the day of the week on which we were born. But as a naturopath, I knew that conventional medicine often took years to catch up with what holistic healers and ancient practitioners had known or used to treat patients for decades or even centuries.

The Gift of Inflammation and Why Your Seven-Day Cycle Matters So Much

After months of conducting research, talking with doctors, and reading all the scientific studies I could find, I felt like I had stumbled on a secret that would upend everything we knew in medicine. The seven-day inflammation-detoxification cycle isn't just an interesting observation on what happens in the body: Inflammation and your body's ability to clear it are the two biggest factors that drive disease, whether we get sick or not, and how we feel on a daily basis. Let me explain.

To understand your seven-day cycle, you first have to know something about inflammation. Acute inflammation occurs anytime you get sick or sustain some type of injury or infection. When that happens, your immune system dispatches an army of white blood cells to the area to help heal the problem. This is a good thing. Without acute inflammation, your body wouldn't be able to recover from a sprained ankle, cut, bug bite, the flu, the common cold, strep throat, or any other injury or illness.

But there's another type of inflammation that isn't so beneficial for your body. Chronic inflammation occurs when your immune system is unable to consistently reduce acute inflammation and/or you're exposed to too many toxins like sugar, cigarette smoke, alcohol, pollution, and/or other chemical irritants in our food and environment. You can also develop chronic inflammation from too much stress, too little sleep, or too much body fat. Since most Americans are stressed, sleep-deprived, and overfed, most of us also have some degree of chronic inflammation.

That's a problem, too: Compared to acute inflammation, which is sudden, temporary, and beneficial, chronic inflammation is slower acting, long-lasting, and detrimental. This can cause tissue damage, genetic changes, and other effects over years that can lead to chronic diseases like cancer, heart disease, diabetes, Alzheimer's, and arthritis. Chronic inflammation can also cause weight gain, fatigue, poor digestion, premature skin aging, joint pain, muscle weakness, depression, brain fog, and a host of other physical, mental, and emotional symptoms.

There's one more type of inflammation that's less understood—and that's the kind your body produces every week as part of its seven-day inflammation-detoxification cycle. Similar to how trees form growth rings in living wood as part of their development and healing process, your body uses your seven-day cycle to grow and heal. Here's how that works.

Every week, your body creates new cells, repairs old ones, and speeds nutrients to your organs, muscles, and other tissues. These are natural, healthy processes you need to grow and heal. But all this cellular activity takes work, which produces byproducts and cellular trash, creating hormones, proteins, and waste that build up in the body and eventually cause inflammation. This inflammation peaks one day every week, which is what I saw in the blood work of all my patients over a decade ago—and what I've seen in every single one of the hundreds of patients I've treated since.

But the body's inflammation levels don't stay sky-high forever—if they did, you wouldn't survive. Similar to how your body has a process to grow and heal, it also has a mechanism to survive that growth and healing: detoxification. Every week, your body breaks down and excretes the excess chemicals that cause your weekly inflammation surge. This is what I call the Cleanse, a two-day detoxification burst that restores the body back to baseline before the entire cycle can start again. During the Cleanse, your kidneys, liver, and lymphatic system—a network of organs, lymph nodes, and lymphatic vessels that acts like a sewer system to help your blood clear toxins from the body—do most of the work, removing the chemicals that are causing inflammation, primarily through urine and feces.

You know that trees keep score of their trauma and growth in the concentric rings in their trunks. They also communicate disease and warnings of drought and other ailments to surrounding flora and fauna through their roots. Similarly, our bodies transmit specific information through our cells, following our natural seven-day cycle.

To help you make sense of this cycle, think of it like repairing and cleaning your house. If you're a homeowner, you know that you have to make regular repairs and clean consistently in order to keep your home comfortable and safe. At the same time, repairing and cleaning takes labor—you'll get dirty and sweaty while doing so and have to take a shower afterward, just like your body labors to create, repair, and restore cells. What's more, when you clean your home, you'll produce trash as you wipe down floors, dust up rooms, touch up walls, and replace any broken appliances or furniture. And you'll have to get rid of this trash or you'll defeat the entire purpose of restoring and cleaning your home in the first place.

The same thing happens in our bodies, which also need regular repairing and cleaning. And similar to what happens when you do a thorough round of spring-cleaning, your body has to use some internal elbow grease and sweat to grow and heal, creating toxins and trash that it has to throw out to stay healthy.

Another way to look at it is this: If you like to lift weights or work out, you're likely familiar with the body's cycle of muscle growth and rest, when tissue has to tear itself in order to build back up stronger and more efficient. The toned muscles we see in the mirror are only indicative of what is happening deep below the surface on a cellular level.

In other words, your body is programmed to grow, heal, and survive—that's what our seven-day inflammation-detoxification cycle is all about. It's your body's gift that keeps on giving, week after week after week, to help make you healthy and whole.

But there's another way that your inflammation-detoxification cycle is a gift: When you know that there are days when inflammation is naturally highest in your body, you can do everything possible, physically, mentally, and emotionally, to reduce your exposure to other inflammation triggers, preventing the kind of chronic inflammation that can cause troubling symptoms, low energy, and lead to illness and disease. Similarly, when you know your body is busy detoxifying, getting rid of the kind of chemicals that cause inflammation, you can do everything possible to encourage it, helping your body break down and eliminate other kinds of inflammation in the process that may be making you sick or causing you to suffer certain symptoms or otherwise feel less than optimal. Let's take a look at how that works.

Using Your Seven-Day Cycle to Your Advantage

Learning about your seven-day inflammation-detoxification cycle is like getting handed the universe's instruction manual for your body: You know exactly what's happening biologically in your body on a weekly basis, when you're most prone to illness because of high inflammation, and when you need to support your body's detoxification process. In other words, our seven-day cycle is the ultimate form of chronomedicine we can each use to help our bodies heal.

By using your seven-day cycle, you can time what you do on a daily basis—how you eat and exercise, when you travel or stress your body in other ways, which medical and self-care treatments you receive and when, how you manage your emotional outlook—to help lower inflammation and speed detoxification. This isn't difficult to do when we break down the seven-day cycle into a day-by-day agenda.

The body's seven-day cycle takes place on a continuum, building inflammation over the course of the week before peaking on the seventh day and detoxifying. After studying our seven-day cycle for more than a decade and testing hundreds of patients' blood every day, I also know what happens in the body on a daily basis. Part of this I gleaned from observing my patients closely every day, watching how they acted and hearing them tell me how they felt. Much of the day-to-day details of our seven-day cycle was also intuitive for me. I also looked at how the body is formed in utero and what that process might look like if we have seven days instead of nine months to rebuild and regenerate.

This is how I came to understand that certain processes occur on different days as the body builds toward its weekly inflammation-detoxification climax. These processes, like cell production and altered blood flow, can also impact how you feel, as well as how adeptly you handle physical or psychological stress. With this knowledge, you can tailor your daily actions to support what's going on in your body, as well as in your life at large. For example, you can eat foods that'll help build new healthy cells on the days of the week this process occurs. You can try to schedule a high-pressure presentation when you know you're most likely to have optimal focus. You can avoid traveling when you know your body needs to recover or opt to do an intense workout on the days when you know your body will perform best.

In short, you can sync your daily activities with your seven-day cycle to improve your work, interpersonal relationships, nutrition, fitness, and day-to-day well-being. Since the same things happen inside the body the same days of the week, week after week, it's easy to learn your body's biological calendar. And once you know it, it's there with you for life to use as a tool whenever you want to boost your health, energy, and overall well-being.

A Daily Snapshot of Your Seven-Day Cycle

To help you understand the body's seven-day inflammation-detoxification cycle and what takes place biologically inside us on a daily basis, let's break it down into two stages. Stage One occurs over the first five days of the cycle, which I refer to as your Days One through Five. This is when the body recovers, repairs, and rebuilds by creating new cells, increasing blood and nutrient flow, and actively working to mend the body. Inflammation is low and only increases slightly on Day Five as hormones, proteins, waste products, and other byproducts of your body's repair work begin to build. In general, most people feel well during Stage One, with more energy, focus, and emotional resiliency, and are able to travel and exercise without feeling sapped or risking injury. You're more likely also to respond well to most kinds of self-care and medical treatment.

Stage Two, which takes place over your Days Six and Seven, is when inflammation peaks and the Cleanse takes places, as your body tries to purge all the hormones, proteins, cellular waste, and other chemicals created by cell renewal and repair over Stage One. During this time, most people have lower energy and focus and less emotional resiliency, may feel irritable or fatigued, aren't able to travel or exercise without it impacting their well-being, and generally don't respond as well to many types of self-care and medical treatment. The results of diagnostic testing done on Days Six and Seven may also be skewed due to high levels of inflammatory markers like C-reactive protein.

In short, the first five days of our seven-day cycle are the body's time to grow and heal; the last two days are when we're inflamed and inundated by the detoxification process. Both stages are imperative for our health and survival and complement each other: Without Stage Two, you couldn't endure Stage One, and vice versa.

In addition, each day in our seven-day cycle follows a specific agenda that affects our physical, mental, and emotional health and function:

Day One: Recover. Day One, which is the day after the day of the week when you were born, is when your body recovers physiologically from the inflammation and detoxification of Days Six and Seven. You may feel a little tired today, especially if your body is holding on to any leftover hormones, protein, cellular waste, and other chemicals it still needs to break down and excrete.

Otherwise, you'll likely feel an acute sense of calm on Day One, as though you've just weathered a major storm—which you have from a physiological standpoint—and all the lightning, thunder, wind, and rain have now cleared. This feeling is reflected biologically in your body, which begins to increase production of the feel-good chemical serotonin today. After two days of intense work, your stomach starts to settle and heal, which helps you feel less bloated than you likely did on Days Six and Seven. Your levels of the stress hormone cortisol, along with estrogen and testosterone, also begin to reregulate, making you feel more emotionally balanced and less tense than you did the past two days.

Day One is a good day to plan and organize but not necessarily to do, since you're still recovering from high inflammation and the Cleanse. This means you'll also want to try to avoid any stressful situations or strenuous activity that might interfere with your recovery. But Day One is an ideal time to set new intentions: As the start of your seven-day cycle, any intention you set today has a better chance of lasting the entire week. The key concept here is observation for inspired action. Today, you have a clean-slate mentality, without any of the heavy, toxic burdens that can lead to feelings of aggression or restlessness—your liver got rid of that on Day Seven. Use your mentality wisely, as the energy you choose to adopt today can last with you all week.

Day Two: Resettle. After a twenty-four-hour recovery period, your body returns to control mode today, using Day Two to maintain a healthy baseline. Out of all days of the week, this is when inflammation levels are lowest—your body has cleared all the excess hormones, proteins, cellular waste, and other chemicals from Days Six and Seven and isn't actively creating, restoring, or rebuilding anything that would create new hormones, proteins, cellular waste, or other inflammatory chemicals. With your blood largely free of these inflammatory markers, there's more room for oxygen, making Day Two the time of the week when your blood is the most oxygenated.

Due to all this highly oxygenated blood flow to the brain and lower inflammation levels, most people have more mental focus and clarity on Day Two than they do the rest of the week. This makes today ideal to give a high-pressure presentation, take a mentally challenging test, or have a difficult conversation with a boss, colleague, spouse, or loved one. If you like to run or weight lift, doing so today when your blood is highly oxygenated can improve your performance while any inflammation sparked by these activities won't overwhelm your body.

Day Three: Restore. After taking a day to recover and another one to resettle, your body is ready to get back to work on Day Three and does so by creating new stem cells, which are the body's basic cells from which all other cells are made. Your body also creates new red blood cells today, which helps to increase your circulation and get nutrients to any of your organs or other tissues that need support. The body also manufactures new white blood cells today, helping to boost your overall immunity.

With increased blood flow and nutrition, you should feel an energizing calm on Day Three. While you had plenty of mental clarity on Day Two, you'll be better able to turn that clarity into action today. This makes Day Three ideal to attack any projects, tasks, or chores you've been putting off, as well as to do any type of interval training or other intense exercise for which improved circulation and nutrition will boost performance and lower recovery times. You'll want to prioritize eating more nutrient-dense foods like almonds and spinach to help keep your blood well-stocked in the nutrients it needs to deliver to different organs, muscles, and other tissues.

Day Four: Rebuild. On Day Four, after a full twenty-four hours of nutrient resupply, your body is ready to rebuild. It does so by turning all those stem cells created on Day Three into specialized cells that it uses to repair muscle, fortify bone, and rebuild your major organs, including your heart and liver. Any specialized cells that aren't used to plug organs, muscles, and bones are sent to fortify your skin, hair, and nails.

Because your body is in an active state of rebuilding today, you'll likely feel more complete and whole, one with the world inside and around you. For many of my patients, Day Four is the day of the week when they feel their best, physically, mentally, and emotionally. The body has had three days to recover, resettle, and restore, and now you feel calm, content, and satisfied. This makes Day Four ideal to socialize—you're more confident and complete—and to make big decisions, since you'll be doing so from a more mentally and emotionally stable place. Prioritizing high-protein foods like salmon and eggs will help your body build back stronger tissue, while getting acupuncture on Day Four can help any new energy meridians become part of your permanent architecture. Similar to recovering from an illness or hard workout, your appetite may also rally today, so make sure to consciously choose foods that represent your desire to nourish and replenish your cells and whole health.

Day Five: Prepare. Day Five is when all the hormones, proteins, and cellular waste created by or used in helping your body repair, restore, and rebuild begin to increase your inflammation levels. The body knows this from a biological standpoint: Just like it anticipates our circadian rhythms by increasing cortisol in the morning and the sleep hormone melatonin at night, the body also anticipates our circaseptan rhythms, activating the central nervous system and immune system and putting its army of pain receptors and white blood cells on high alert. The liver begins to produce more bile, which helps eliminate waste products and toxins through feces. Toward the end of Day Five, your kidneys kick into gear, increasing how much blood they filter and turning excess waste into urine. You also begin to produce more cortisol and C-reactive protein—both inflammatory markers—as the day goes on.

It's not all about inflammation today, however. After restoring and rebuilding all your internal organs, the body also turns its attention to your skin today, as your skin cells regenerate. Because your skin is in the process of regeneration and healing, Day Five is ideal for any type of facial or cosmetic treatment.

You'll still have plenty of energy on Day Five, but you may feel a little more sensitive or apprehensive, as your body prepares for the following days. This makes today a good time to prepare for things in your own life, too, and take care of any loose ends. You may want to scale back on the intensity of your exercise, focusing on low-impact activities like swimming or yoga that won't increase inflammation like intense or high-impact exercise will.

Stage Two: The Last Two Days of the Week

Day Six: Flush. The storm is finally here, as your body surges in inflammation and begins the Cleanse. Levels of the stress hormone cortisol and C-reactive protein continue to increase on Day Six, along with interferons, which are proteins secreted by your immune cells in response to viruses and infection. Your kidneys, which start to clean more blood on Day Five, pick up the pace on Day Six, filtering and flushing more through urine than they will all week—why you'll be thirstier and likely have to make more trips to the bathroom today. Activity in your liver and lymphatic system also increases today, as both begin to detoxify, eventually taking over the job from the kidneys on Day Seven.

These physiological processes are necessary to help your body detoxify, but they do come at a cost: With higher levels of inflammation and detoxification activity, you'll likely feel a little tired and sluggish today, perhaps even foggy, irritable, or overly sensitive. This may be similar to how you feel when you're coming down with something—you might be somewhat agitated, perhaps even a bit achy. Many patients also tell me they feel frustrated on Day Six, as though they can't get out of their own way, which makes sense: Your body is literally tripping up on its own inflammation and trying to get rid of it.

At the same time, you can lean into what's happening in your body today by staying hydrated, helping your kidneys filter and flush as much as possible. Think about how you can avoid stressful situations that are likely to raise cortisol and blood pressure, which will slow kidney function. Instead, look for ways to slow things down for yourself a little—for instance, soaking in a float tank or taking a bath with Epsom salts will help balance your electrolyte levels and support your kidneys, while gentle movements like tai chi or water aerobics will increase lymph movement and lower cortisol.

Day Seven: Rebirth. Day Seven is the most critical in your seven-day cycle. This is when your body is most inflamed and every inflammatory chemical spikes, including cortisol, estrogen, interferons, cellular waste, and viral debris. What you do on Day Seven has a big impact on your overall health, depending on whether you work with your body to lower inflammation or work against it by doing things that increase your inflammatory load.

Day Seven is also when most of the Cleanse occurs and when your body, particularly your liver and lymphatic system, goes into overdrive to get rid of its weekly inflammation. What you do today will determine the shape of your next seven-day cycle. You can help your body detoxify everything possible by taking it easy and actively seeking out gentle treatments. Or you could wind up impairing the process, opening up the floodgates for inflammation to remain in the body and lead to possible ailments, illness, and disease.

If you give your liver the necessary nutritional support and space it needs today to detoxify fully from its preceding six-day toxic burden, it can also begin to process and excrete underlying chronic inflammation and cellular debris. This is where the real magic happens, when you have the chance to take your body out of a state of catabolic reaction, when metabolic changes occur in individual cells, to steady-state homeostasis, when your entire body starts to normalize and maintain a healthy baseline without being overwhelmed by chronic inflammation. It's like your body is a car and you can either use the automatic brakes to avoid hitting something or pull the emergency brake and hope it works to stop you.

As for your energy and emotional well-being, Day Seven can be a bit of a roller-coaster ride. You may wake up feeling like you've been hit by a truck or revved up and ready to go. Both are natural as your body copes with inflammation, which can cause fatigue, along with intense detoxification, which can boost energy and even trigger feelings of elation. No matter what you feel, it's important to relax, prioritize healthy foods, stay hydrated, and get enough sleep so you can help support your liver and lymphatic system without adding more inflammation. Journaling can also help you identify and work through any emotions excavated by the Cleanse.

The Day Seven Dilemma: When and How Illness Occurs

Day Seven is also critical because it's when illness is most likely to occur in the body on a biological and cellular level. As inflammation peaks, every cell, tissue, and organ inside you fights back while your liver and lymphatic system try to keep pace, working to detoxify that inflammation. All this effort and inflammation make your body more vulnerable than any other time during the week, and it's easier for illness to slip in and take a seat on Day Seven. It's also easier for any existing symptoms or ailments you have to intensify after Day Seven if the liver and lymphatic system are unable to eliminate weekly inflammation.

There's something else happening inside your body today: As the Cleanse scours for inflammatory chemicals and eliminates them from your cells, the process can stir up painful emotions or memories that live inside the body (more on this in later chapters). So not only are you more vulnerable physically on Day Seven, you're also more vulnerable emotionally. You're more likely to be tired, irritable, and sensitive, so any unpleasant events, conversations, thoughts, or feelings that occur today may take a bigger toll or leave a longer-lasting impression on you.

According to the latest research, human emotions and memories are manifested physically, by our cells and organs, on a visceral, biological level. A 2013 landmark study by a team of Finnish researchers, for example, found that human beings feel the same emotions in the same parts of the body over and over again, regardless of their sex, age, culture, or how their language expresses feelings (e.g., Americans use the phrase "butterflies in the stomach" to describe anxiety or nervousness).[5]

More important, many Western medical doctors and traditional Chinese medicine practitioners also believe that human beings somatize past traumas, meaning we store bad events and incidents that have happened to us in our bodies, oftentimes for years, because our brains can't deal with them.[6] These traumas, which researchers estimate 70 percent of all Americans experience, can include everything from rape, abuse, and death in the family to a bad breakup, the pivotal loss of a job, or persistent illness.[7] We'll talk more about how emotions live in the body and affect our health in chapter 5.

While Day Seven is a vulnerable time for a number of reasons, you have the power to protect your body and prevent new illnesses, existing ailments, or old emotions from taking a deeper seat inside your cells. This power comes from leaning into your seven-day cycle and working with your body to lower inflammation and purge as much of the bad stuff as possible. In other words, the decisions you make about your health all week can either help you prevent illness or increase the possibility that inflammation, old illness, and trauma will remain in your body after Day Seven. Every day, you wake up with the ability to make choices that will improve your health, energy, and ability to heal. All you have to do is start listening to the ancient wisdom your body has been following since the day you were born.

YOUR BIRTHDAY
AND THE PROTOCOL

CHAPTER 3

T he body's seven-day inflammation-detoxification cycle is universal: Every person on the planet has the same circaseptan rhythms, which connect us all with one another and with the universe at large. We ebb and flow with our circaseptan rhythms, just like the earth, moon, sun, and seas do, forming a harmonious master musical piece of life.

While we all have the same seven-day cycle, when that cycle occurs inside each of us is unique, based on our personal biology. We each have a different day of the week when we're most inflamed, vulnerable to illness, and experience the Cleanse. What's happening in your body on a Monday or Friday may not be the same as what's happening inside your spouse, mother, sister, cousin, colleague, or a stranger you meet on the street.

In chapters 1 and 2, I explained how the day of the week on which you were born is the key to your own seven-day cycle. In the midst of the universal, there is this deeply individual adaptation that was assigned to you, at your moment of birth. Now I want to explain why your birthday is so important so you can personalize the Protocol and start changing your life, one week at a time.

Why and How We Relive the Alchemy of Birth Each Week

Your seven-day cycle didn't start when you were conceived, nor did it start when you were in the womb. Before you were born, you were dependent on your mother for all life's biological processes, including respiration, nutrition, growth, and movement. Your rhythms were her rhythms, and everything she did affected what occurred inside you.

But the moment you were born, the universe pushed the "start button" on your seven-day cycle. You were no longer dependent on your mother to breathe, eat, grow, move, and excrete—you had to perform all these functions on your own in order to survive. It was time to start your own biological life processes. This may make you think the day of the week on which you were born is your Day One. But it's not: The day of the week that you were born is your Day Seven—and it was the biggest and most important day of your life.

Here's what happened. On the day you were born, Little Newborn You went from the warm, quiet, dark, cozy comfort of your mother's womb into the loud, bright world. All of a sudden, you were looking at glaring fluorescent lights and hearing sharp, loud noises. For the first time, you felt oxygen whooshing on your skin and trying to batter down into your respiratory tract and little lungs. This amounted to sudden shock, as you traded the calm, homeostatic environment of your mother's womb for the chaotic, noisy, all-systems-go environment of the real world.

The shock of this transition cannot be understated. It's as though someone took you out of a quiet meditation room where you'd been living peacefully for nine months and suddenly shoved you into a Metallica concert during the final encore—it's a massive amount of stress for the body to handle. Despite the advances in modern medicine and birthing practices that are constantly evolving, one million babies continue to die every year worldwide on the day they are born.[1] This was your make-or-break moment as a living creature—and your body had to do everything it could to make sure you made it.

As soon as you left the womb, all your body's biological systems switched to *go*. Your lungs had to expand, your muscles had to move, and your sensory organs had to work, as your eyes opened to receive light, and you began to smell, hear, and feel. Your immune system had to start working, and you immediately began looking for food in order to survive—why newborns who don't breastfeed in the first hour after birth have a 41 percent lower chance of survival.[2] At the same time, you also had to excrete to get rid of the toxins that infants accumulate in the womb—why a baby's first poop is a tarry and dark green with old cells, mucus, bile, and other waste products.

Triggering all these biological processes at the same time placed an incredible degree of stress on your body. This, in turn, generated a ton of inflammation everywhere, as your body raced to make sure that everything was working at the same time. This stress was combined with the shock of birth itself, as your nervous system initiated its fight-or-flight response for the first time, flooding Little Newborn You with cortisol and other hormones, neurotransmitters, and waste byproducts. While the moments after a baby's birth may seem peaceful if you're the mother or an observer in the room, a newborn is dealing with astronomically high levels of stress hormones. All these chemicals increase inflammation, which surged inside you the day you were born.

Since your body can't survive sky-high inflammation levels for long, Little Newborn You initiated the best and only biological process the body has to get rid of all the excess chemicals surging inside you: You detoxified, using your newborn kidneys, liver, and lymphatic system to remove as many toxins as possible created by the process of birth and your first fight for survival. This detoxification lasted about a day, taking up the first full twenty-four hours of your life.

Once your body had cleared out all the chemicals causing inflammation, Little Newborn You began to calm down and heal from the trauma of your birth. In fact, the day after your birth was your biggest time ever of recovery. If you're a parent, you've likely witnessed this firsthand, watching your highly agitated and colicky baby on the day they were born transform into a creature the next day who simply wants to sleep, eat, and exist.

Over the course of the next several days, Little Newborn You's energy increased as your body began the process of repairing and growing. As your body created new cells, restored nutrition to various organs and other tissues, and built the areas inside you that would ensure your continued health and survival, it also created a ton of hormones, proteins, cellular waste, and other chemicals that slowly began to increase. These chemicals, in excess, eventually caused your inflammation to peak so that your little body had to initiate another detoxification round, similar to the day you were born, to get rid of that inflammation. This is how your body's seven-day inflammation-detoxification cycle began, with the trauma of your birth sparking the inflammation peak and Cleanse that takes place on Day Seven.

Why would our bodies want to repeat the trauma of our birth, which is the most traumatic physical event we've ever endured?

For that answer, just look at basic biology. When a living creature discovers a process that allows it to survive, it tries to repeat that process over and over again in order to ensure its continued survival. The body essentially thinks to itself, *Wow, I almost died, but I didn't. I should keep doing whatever I did to survive because it worked.*

Your body repeats other biological traumas to ensure its survival, too. For example, when you're exposed to a virus, your body develops antibodies to make sure you're able to fight that virus for years to come, even if you're never exposed again. Similarly, your body initiates its fight-or-flight response every time you're faced with something potentially harmful or traumatic, even though doing so takes a toll on your health, increasing cortisol and other inflammatory markers.

While the idea of repeating trauma may sound like a bad thing, it's actually a beautiful gift. Repeating events is what establishes our master circaseptan rhythm and the seven-day inflammation-detoxification cycle inside us all that we can use to begin to overhaul health and energy in just one week's time.

The Protocol: Turning the Trauma of Birth into Optimal Health and Well-Being

Using your seven-day cycle to unlock optimal health starts with something called the Protocol, a tool I've been using with patients and celebrity clients for years to help them overhaul their energy, overcome disease and other ailments, prevent illness, discover greater emotional balance and well-being, and achieve new heights in health and happiness. Relying on the knowledge of what happens in the body every day during the seven-day cycle, the Protocol combines the use of targeted nutrition, dietary supplements, exercise recommendations, suggested lifestyle tweaks, stress-management behaviors, emotional maintenance, and the smart timing of medical and self-care treatments to help lower inflammation and increase your body's detoxification process. The less inflammation you have and the more you can eliminate through the Cleanse each week, the healthier you'll be, physically, mentally, emotionally, and spiritually.

In this book, I will give you the specific tools to help you regenerate and repair your body's healing systems. Beyond that, I will also show you the direct pain-body connection you can access in order to release the emotional source of disease that may be smoldering inside you. Finally, I will teach you everything you need to know about how to adopt the Protocol to get the results you want, whether you follow the plan for just one week's time or want to lean into your seven-day cycle for as long as you can.

Here's one thing to know about the Protocol: If you google the plan or ask your doctor about it, you won't find any answers. The Protocol is what I created after discovering the existence of our seven-day cycle to help hundreds of patients lean into the body's natural biorhythms and the ancient wisdom that can help us all heal. It's a preventative strategy as much as a treatment plan, meaning it can prevent minor issues like premature aging, weight gain, and skin conditions as much as it can help treat chronic diseases like cancer, diabetes, and Alzheimer's.

I believe we're entering a new phase of medicine that will be strongly rooted in preventative care rather than in acute care. This shift will mark a significant change in how Western health care currently operates. Today, conventional Western medicine is primarily focused on saving the lives of the seriously sick rather than preventing the kind of chronic disease that causes people to get sick in the first place. Conventional doctors tend to isolate and treat disease, rather than take a holistic view of a patient's entire body. To me, that is the equivalent of trying to control the ocean's tides by ignoring the moon. Part of the reason for this is historical: Saving lives centuries ago took precedent over preventing diseases that weren't well understood. Another reason, unfortunately, is money: Chronic disease and the acute care required to treat it are extremely lucrative, obviating the incentive to focus on the kind of interventions and treatments needed to help us stay healthy and avoid inflammation in the first place.

What this means is that you can't necessarily rely on conventional medicine to help you prevent disease or achieve any kind of optimal health. It's up to you to take control of and responsibility for your own health and well-being. This became even more obvious during the coronavirus pandemic, when people with chronic illnesses like obesity, diabetes, and high blood pressure were more likely to get seriously sick or die from COVID-19. While these conditions may not have been an instant death sentence in the past, all it took was one virus to show the world we need to be as healthy as possible and that it's up to each of us to do so, shoring up our own physical well-being before the next virus or other threat emerges.

Compared to conventional medicine, naturopathic medical practices exist to help prevent disease and treat the whole body. They target the root causes of ailments instead of simply suppressing a certain symptom or waiting until a patient develops an illness or gets seriously sick to address the problem. This means that if you want to prevent disease, feel good, and discover what optimal health feels like without having to get sick first, you may have to think outside the box and look beyond conventional medicine. This may mean considering ideas that aren't backed by conventional science or that may make you uncomfortable at first because you've never heard of or seen them in practice. But if COVID-19 taught us anything, it's that getting uncomfortable is sometimes the only way to discover transformative things about our health, our bodies, and what we need to do to live better.

After I discovered the body's seven-day inflammation-detoxification cycle, I knew I had to do something to help my patients, many of whom were facing serious or terminal illnesses, take advantage of this master circaseptan rhythm and leverage chronomedicine to help improve their health. I started with the centerpiece of our seven-day cycle—Day Seven—since it's the day when inflammation peaks and detoxification occurs in the body. After that, I worked backward to figure out how to arrange the puzzle pieces of what people can do on a daily basis so that their lives, diet, and habits could best support what was happening inside their bodies on Day Seven, physically, emotionally, and spiritually. Suddenly, I had a plan for what my patients could do each day of the week to best support Day Seven and the Cleanse.

Using the Protocol, I could tell when any medical treatment or complementary therapy would be the most beneficial or effective for someone based on his or her seven-day cycle. I stopped drawing blood from my patients on their Day Seven, as well as the day before (Day Six) and day after (Day One), when I knew their inflammation levels would be elevated because of the Cleanse and their results would likely be an inaccurate reflection of what was really going on. In addition, I recommended no one have surgery or any other invasive procedures Days Six and Seven when their bodies would have to struggle to cope with more inflammation, their recovery times would be slower, and the procedures might not be as effective due to high inflammation. For those patients who had chemotherapy, I suggested they schedule the treatment for Day Five when their bodies would still be able to absorb the medication, yet they'd also start detoxifying the next day (Day Six), so the toxic stuff wouldn't say in their system too long. I advised patients to receive acupuncture on Day Four, when the body rebuilds and can best incorporate any new energy patterns into its permanent infrastructure. If ice baths or hot saunas were someone's thing, I wanted my patients to do so on their Day Three, when I knew the boost in nutrient delivery in the body would make either therapy more advantageous.

In short, this was chronomedicine at its best: I was able to personalize medical treatment and therapy to a patient's individual timetable so that the treatments would actually work. I was leveraging a practice that researchers have called "medicine's secret ingredient"[3] and "a necessary concept to manage human diseases"[4] but which hardly any doctors use because it takes time, effort, and, most critical, understanding. I believe the Protocol is the ultimate form of chronomedicine, and it's yours right now to learn, adopt, and use to take control of your health for years to come.

But the Protocol isn't just about timing your medical treatments and therapies with your seven-day cycle; it's about finally aligning with your body's oldest and most original state of truth and balance. When you get in touch with your natural biorhythms, you start to have intimate conversations with your body and mind through the eyes of your emotion and spirit. This journey isn't a quick fix—it's a pathway to reconnection, lasting wisdom, and transformation from the inside out.

Soon after I discovered the body's master circaseptan rhythm, I created a targeted supplement regimen for patients that uses plant-based medicine to help drive down the inflammation building in their bodies Days One through Five while increasing the detoxification process Days Six and Seven. This means taking no other supplements Days Six and Seven that don't support detoxification, as those nutrients will just be purged from the body as part of the Cleanse—money down the toilet, literally. While I didn't and still don't mandate that patients take supplements, I tell them that doing so can make a huge difference to their health and how they feel on a daily basis.

In the years since discovering the body's seven-day cycle, I've also created a healthy eating plan as part of the Protocol to help patients consume the foods that will best support what's going on in their bodies. It's similar to taking certain supplements on certain days: When you eat the right foods at the right times, it will help your body lower inflammation, create new cells, build new tissue, heal, and better detoxify. For example, I want to encourage you to eat foods like spinach, cranberries, and garlic on Day One to increase lymphatic drainage so that your body can clear any leftover hormones, proteins, cellular waste, and other inflammatory chemicals. But on Day Two, when your body returns to baseline, you'll want to prioritize foods that lower your inflammatory set point so that you're starting from a decreased place of inflammation for the week—foods like broccoli, green tea, and reishi mushrooms. Similarly, on Day Three, the best way that you can support your body is by eating foods that are nutrient dense, packed with vitamins, minerals, antioxidants, and healthy fats, since your body restores nutrition to all your organs, muscles, and other tissues on this day.

Just like nutrition, exercise plays a part in the Protocol, as being active can help you either increase or decrease your body's inflammatory load and detoxification activity. Choosing to do fluid movements like yoga, tai chi, and swimming on Day One, for example, won't increase your inflammation when your body is trying to recover but can stimulate your lymphatic system to get rid of any inflammatory toxins leftover from the Cleanse. Several days later, though, on Day Three, you'll want to take advantage of the fact that your circulatory system is in high gear and your muscles and joints are bathed in blood and nutrients to do a race or high-intensity interval training (HIIT). Similarly, you'll want to avoid intense workouts on Days One, Six, and Seven, when your body has high levels of inflammation, which intense exercise can exacerbate, increasing the risk of injury and impairing your detoxification process.

You can also use the Protocol to pace out the rest of your life. When it's possible, you can time a wide variety of activities based on when your body is best up to the task. For instance, you can aim to travel on Days Two through Four, when you have the most energy and the least inflammation. You can also try to attack big projects on Days Two to Four, when your mental focus and motivation are highest, thanks to low inflammation and increased blood flow. Schedule a first date or big social function on Day Four in particular, when you're most likely to feel confident and complete, thanks to the body's active rebuilding process. That's also when you'll want to make high-risk decisions, as you'll be more mentally and emotionally stable than you'll be all week. Day Five is ideal for taking care of loose ends before inflammation and detoxification sap your energy, while Day One—the start of your seven-day cycle—is great to set goals or intentions for the rest of the week. Days Six and Seven are the best time to give yourself permission to relax while you stay open to epiphanies, as the Cleanse can often excavate old emotions and amazing new ideas. In short, every day of the week has an exciting component, and getting tuned in to the Protocol can help you appreciate each day and maximize every moment.

Understanding the Protocol also provides insight into why you're more tired, irritable, or sensitive one day, while you may feel serene and optimistic the next. This can help you lean into these feelings and accept them, working with your body to nourish your emotional outlook rather than fearing or trying to fight against it.

Benefits of the Protocol

Remember those twenty-five patients who helped me discover the presence of the body's seven-day cycle? The same ones I blood-tested every day for three months? This group was the first to follow the Protocol—and after just three months on the plan, all twenty-five experienced some incredible benefits. Two with terminal illness, including Katie, went into remission—something that conventional health care, with all its toxic medications and invasive operations, had never been able to accomplish for these patients. It blew my mind to see these two patients in relative unison become disease-free of conditions like cancer after other doctors had written them off as untreatable, all because they had altered their habits to live by the Protocol.

But the benefits went far beyond terminal illness. All the other patients in my initial research group were able to cure or reverse the ailments that caused them to make appointments with me in the first place—in some instances, they had battled these health issues for years. Many also lost weight, started sleeping better, had more balanced energy, experienced less bloating and indigestion, and had fewer mood swings or feelings of anger, anxiety, or sadness.

Shortly after this, I started following the Protocol, too. I wanted to experience the benefits, but I also wanted to know what the plan would do for someone who wasn't sick or didn't have any existing health issues. For much of my life, I had always dreaded Mondays and never understood why. I assumed it was because Monday starts the workweek, yet even when I've had jobs I've loved and couldn't wait to get into the office, Mondays still seemed more laborious, like I couldn't get out of bed, no matter how excited I might have been for the day. When I started using the Protocol and realized my Day Seven—the day of the week when I was born—is Monday, I understood why I didn't like Mondays, and I started giving myself permission to take it a little easier. This made a huge difference in my energy levels the rest of the week: Leaning into my inflammation and detoxification activity gave my body the time-out it needed to get rid of more inflammatory chemicals and recover faster from the process.

After a few months on the Protocol, I experienced some of the same transformation my patients had. I was sleeping better, my digestion had improved, and my hair, skin, and nails were looking healthier. The headaches I occasionally had were now almost nonexistent, and I felt more positive, grounded, and even happier. I was more aligned, balanced, and intentional about every aspect of my life, including my movements, my relationships, even the foods I chose to eat. I felt more present in my body, like I had finally fallen in step with what was going on inside me and driving me forward. This is the beauty of the Protocol: It doesn't matter if you're suffering from a major illness, a minor ailment, or simply wanting to optimize your health.

Slash the Kind of Inflammation That Causes Most Health Issues, Illnesses, and Disease

At the heart of it, the benefits of the Protocol are the result of lowering inflammation and improving detoxification. Let's take a closer look.

When you adopt the Protocol, you do three things that help reduce inflammation drastically:

1. You eat certain foods, take specific supplements, do targeted activities and exercise, and time medical, self-care, or complementary therapies to help reduce inflammation.
2. You avoid eating certain foods, doing high-intensity exercise, undertaking stressful activities, or receiving more invasive medical, self-care, or complementary therapies when you know they'll raise inflammation at times when the body can't handle it.
3. You actively encourage detoxification on Days Six and Seven, helping your body eliminate more inflammation.

As you know from chapter 2, inflammation is the primary driver of many health issues, illnesses, and diseases, from major conditions like cancer, diabetes, and autoimmune disorders to more minor ailments like eczema, back pain, and weight gain. While weekly increases in inflammation are normal, beneficial, and necessary to trigger the regular detoxification we need to stay healthy, when you incur too much chronic inflammation over time, it forces your immune system to be always on alert,[5] lessening its ability to prevent other ailments and interfering with the optimal function of other systems in your body, including your metabolism, blood sugar regulation, cell production, ability to repair and heal tissue, cognitive function, and microbiome—the essential community of bacteria in the gut that influence mood, digestion, metabolism, and a host of other critical faculties.

Whether you already have a health condition or simply want to prevent disease, weight gain, and all the other ailments associated with inflammation, doing everything possible to reduce your inflammatory load is key. You can reduce inflammation with diet, exercise, sleep, and stress management, but no matter how healthy you eat or how much sleep or exercise you get, if you're out of sync with your body's clock, inflammation can overwhelm your system and cause you to be sick—which is why people who follow healthy lifestyles can still be overweight, be plagued by unpleasant symptoms, and/or develop chronic disease. Scientists have already proven what can happen when you disrupt your circadian rhythms by eating, sleeping, exercising, and taking on certain activities that defy the body's twenty-four-hour clock: You dysregulate the immune system and cause the kind of chronic inflammation that can lead to disease symptoms and disease itself.[6]

The same happens when you disrupt your master circaseptan rhythm: Your immune system gets overloaded, causing chronic inflammation. The way to prevent this effect, just like getting up with the sun and going to bed at night to stay aligned with your circadian rhythms, is to tune in to that rhythm and do everything you can to live in sync with your seven-day cycle.

Increasing the Body's Ability to Detoxify

There is a lot of discussion these days about detoxification and what we can do to help the body eliminate the toxic buildup from the things we eat, the chemicals we're exposed to every day, the stress we incur, and all the other influences of modern life. But the truth is, expensive juice cleanses and all-day sweat sessions aren't the best way to help your body detox: The body is quite capable of detoxifying itself, as researchers and scientists have stated and shown us over and over again.[7] The body relies primarily on the liver, lymphatic system, and kidneys to filter and flush toxins, including those that cause inflammation, in addition to the skin, immune system, respiratory system, and gut. No amount of green juice, sweat, dietary supplements, or other detox tactics can trigger all these systems to work or work in unison—in fact, sweating too much or taking the wrong kind of nutrients can impair the ability of your liver, lymphatic system, kidneys, and body as a whole to filter and flush.

What we do know about promoting detoxification is that the body undertakes an elimination period once every seven days, getting rid of the inflammatory markers created by cell production and repair that occur over the course of the week. This means that if you want to help your body better detoxify, you need to take care of your body—primarily your liver, lymphatic system, and kidneys—during this weekly detoxification burst, or what I call the Cleanse. Adopting science-backed ways to support your liver, lymphatic system, and kidneys on Days Six and Seven will help you get rid of the most toxins possible—not only those responsible for weekly inflammation surges but also the kind of chemicals that may be triggering longer-lasting chronic inflammation that can lead to health issues and illnesses.

Supporting your liver, lymphatic system, and kidneys during the Cleanse will achieve the goals that a lot of fad detoxes promise. Doing this will also help you eliminate harmful viral debris in your body. At any given time, there are approximately 380 trillion viruses living inside you, which is collectively referred to as the human virome.[8] Some are beneficial to the body, but others can be harmful and cause health issues, illness, or outright disease if they remain in the body too long. The body is capable of handling them in its own way, and what you do will either facilitate or interfere with your body's ability to best manage your vast virome.

Lowering your inflammation levels and increasing your body's ability to detoxify has a host of specific physical, mental, and emotional benefits. Here's a quick snapshot of what you can expect to see, think, and feel after seven days of living in sync with your body by following the Protocol:

Physical Benefits of the Protocol

- Improves the health of your internal organs, including your liver, kidneys, heart, lungs, skin, gastrointestinal tract, and reproductive organs
- Reduces the stress hormone cortisol and overall oxidative stress on a cellular level
- Increases energy and stamina by lowering inflammation and cortisol while increasing physical health and function
- Improves digestion and reduces bloating, constipation, acid reflux, and other gastrointestinal symptoms
- Balances hormone production, including estrogen, testosterone, and thyroid hormones
- Lowers your body's overall viral load to help you better fight off and prevent illness
- Prevents bacterial imbalances and boosts the function of your microbiome to improve gut health
- Treats or reverses nutrient deficiencies or problems with nutrient absorption
- Triggers weight loss by lowering inflammation, balancing hormones, improving digestion, reversing nutrient deficiencies, and stimulating metabolism
- Increases stem cell production, boosting the body's ability to grow new cells
- Rejuvenates overall skin health for clearer, younger, fresher skin
- Reduces the frequency and severity of headaches and migraines

- Stimulates hair and nail growth through lower inflammation levels and increased stem cell production
- Improves athletic performance and limits muscle and joint pain, soreness, and weakness

---

The Surprising Beauty Benefits of the Protocol

When you adopt the Protocol, surprising things can happen, including a host of benefits that will transform how you look. Take, for example, one of my patients who had gone prematurely gray in his twenties and was now losing his hair. When I started working with Jason, forty-one, he had tried every prescription medication and over-the-counter regrowth formula on the market. Nothing had worked, and by the time we were introduced, he'd resigned himself to being bald. I immediately put Jason on the Protocol, and fast-forward six months, he was regrowing hair on his head and had even begun sprouting new hair on his chest, which he'd never experienced before.

The Protocol helps you grow and preserve stem cells, or cells that divide into specialized cells to help proliferate and repair hair, nail, bone, muscle, and other tissues in the body. When you adopt the Protocol, you also lower your body's levels of inflammation and toxicity, which helps improve the health of your hair, skin, and nails while also increasing and protecting stem cells. The supplement curcumin, which I recommend everyone who adopts the Protocol take on Days One through Five (see page 66 for more information), also stimulates and protects stem cell production, according to a number of studies.[9]

Using the Protocol to Change Your Life

The Protocol is an intense process of self-discovery, healing, and reinvention. When you start paying attention and listening to your body, you open a whole new door into your body, life, and self that often produces profound emotional effects alongside the mental and physical ones. We'll talk about how to use the Protocol to overhaul your emotional health in chapter 5, but in short, when you change your physical body, you change your mind and the feelings you have there, too—they're all connected.

I see this happen all the time with my patients: When they adopt the Protocol, it forces them to stop, take a breath, and consider how, why, and for what they're living their lives. Patricia, forty-five, for example, started to see me because both of her parents were diabetics, and she was concerned about developing the disease now that she was in middle age. When we began working together, the first thing I did was put her on the Protocol, paying special attention to her diet. We removed both grains and dairy from her overall diet to help lower her inflammation and better manage her blood sugar. In addition, I knew she needed some energetic, psychological, and spiritual work, because she had a lot of fears and preexisting beliefs around diabetes. We talked about these fears and how she could let go of her idea that she would get diabetes—a family history, after all, isn't a diagnosis unless you believe it to be.

We also talked a lot about Patricia's harmful relationship with her father. She hadn't spoken with him in twenty years and had a lot of anger toward him, which was impacting her health. When she finally aligned with her body's biological rhythms and worked toward purging as much as she could on Day Seven—not only her physical traumas but also her emotional ones—she was able to let go of some of the anger toward her father. After three weeks on the Protocol, she called him and made amends. It couldn't have come at a better time: He died a month after the two reconnected.

What Patricia's story shows is that when you start living in sync with your seven-day cycle, other areas of your life can fall into place. With less inflammation, stress, and disease symptoms—and with more mental and emotional stability and clarity—you have the ability and power to start seeing some aspects of your life more clearly and acutely. Your health is your life, and the Protocol is designed to give you a new perspective and understanding of how you, as an individual, tick.

Mental and Emotional Benefits of the Protocol

- Increases cognitive function, including your executive function, which is your ability to plan, organize, manage time, multitask, and focus
- Reduces brain fog and feelings of confusion and mental sluggishness
- Lowers levels of stress and anxiety
- Helps treat and even reverse depression

- Reduces feelings of anger, irritability, frustration, agitation, and aggression
- Increases feelings of alignment and connectedness with your body
- Promotes feelings of being grounded and centered
- Helps you recognize and identify underlying emotions and potential emotional traumas
- Releases emotions that can be trapped in the visceral body
- Stimulates and allows for deeper emotional healing
- Shifts your mental and emotional focus from outward to inward
- Can help you feel less chaotic and more empathetic toward others

Spiritual Benefits of the Protocol

- Can stimulate you to discover and nurture new sides of yourself and your spirit
- Gives you permission to be gentler and more forgiving with yourself
- Allows you to be more present in each and every day
- Initiates or enhances how you communicate with your body
- Can stimulate you to start changing other aspects of your life
- Allows you to understand and experience how everyone has an individual process
- Can help you step into your power and be an advocate for your own health
- Helps you prioritize yourself, in turn creating stronger boundaries with others
- Improves your relationship with yourself, in turn improving your relationship with others
- Can help deepen romantic relationships or help you discover the love you're looking for

MAKING THE PROTOCOL
WORK FOR YOU

CHAPTER 4

The first time I talked with Krista was over the phone. At the time, I had no idea who she was. I just assumed she was another Los Angeles social-ite who, like so many others in the City of Angels, was more than a little obsessed with a jet-set life of parties, continual travel, and red-carpet events.

But days after we first started talking by phone, I received a nondisclosure agreement from Krista's agent. It became clear to me that Krista wasn't just an-other socialite but one of the most legendary actresses in all of Hollywood. When she talked to me about red-carpets events, it wasn't because she was trying to climb the social ladder; she was already on the top and was obligated to attend.

The reason I was speaking with Krista in the first place was because I had helped her daughter, June (who was a fairly famous actress in her own right), overhaul thyroid issues she had been dealing with for months. June was im-pressed with the results and wanted to see if I could help her mother, too.

When I first started working with Krista, she didn't have any distinct health issues per se. But like so many people, she didn't feel great—or as optimally as both she and I knew she could feel. She was often tired and stressed and con-tinually concerned that her lifestyle was taking a big toll on her energy, digestion, and physical appearance. She also traveled a lot, which was adding to her energy drain and increasing her overall stress at the time. She also wanted to see if she could improve her stamina to better withstand the intense spotlight most celeb-rities live under while looking as good as possible for the cameras that trailed her everywhere.

I knew Krista could boost her energy and how well she felt and looked, but in order for her to do so, I needed one critical piece of information: the day of the week on which she was born. Krista was born on a Thursday, which means that was her Day Seven—the day of the week when her body's seven-day inflammation-detoxification cycle peaks over and over again.

Once we knew her body's schedule, we talked about how we could adjust what she did on a daily basis to better line up with her own internal seven-day cycle of inflammation and detoxification. She didn't need to be convinced that the Protocol would work—she had already seen how it had helped her daughter, June—and she immediately started making changes. She started thinking about her body's personal circaseptan rhythms as she made decisions about when and what she ate, when and how she exercised, when she traveled, when and what supplements she took. She considered them as she set her schedule and planned activities.

For example, on the Protocol, Krista began to minimize how often she traveled on Wednesdays and Thursdays—her Days Six and Seven, when we knew her body would already be under duress with a lot of inflammation and detoxification activity. Instead, she tried to book trips whenever possible on Mondays and Tuesdays—her Days Four and Five, when we knew her body would have more circulating nutrition and better immune function. Saturdays and Sundays—her Days Two and Three—were also fine for travel, but she tried to avoid big activities on Fridays, which was her Day One and a good day to take it easy after her body's big inflammation-detoxification surge.

In addition to tweaking her travel schedule, Krista also began taking supplements to help her body better detoxify on Days Six and Seven, when we knew her body would be purging accumulated inflammatory markers and other substances. She also started prioritizing foods that would help her body heal and mitigate inflammation for the first part of her seven-day cycle.

But we didn't just change Krista's lifestyle habits. I also suggested she readjust her mental outlook to better align with what was happening inside her body. For example, since all Krista's stress hormones would be higher on Wednesdays and Thursdays (her Days Six and Seven), I recommended that she take extra care to avoid reading about herself in the press on those days, as she would be more vulnerable to getting upset or potentially overreacting to coverage that felt negative. We talked about how she was more likely to feel calm over the weekends and thereby more open to practicing meditation and mindfulness. I made her aware that she could probably expect to feel a little more tired and irritable on Wednesdays, Thursdays, and even Fridays—that would be important for her to know as she moved through the world. Becoming mindful of when she was likely to be more sensitive allowed her to give herself—and others—a little more grace on those days.

Krista was no stranger to holistic medicine, but she was excited to think about the natural rhythms of her seven-day cycle in a new way.

Just a few weeks after Krista started the Protocol, she called to tell me that her digestion had improved significantly, that she felt less bloated and more comfortable after meals. Moreover, she said she had more energy, as though she'd suddenly gained a pep in her step. She thought her hair and nails were growing faster, stronger, and thicker, and she had even lost a few pounds to boot.

One month later, I got another call: Now eight weeks into the Protocol, Krista was sleeping better, her energy was continuing to increase every day, and she said she was finally waking up feeling well rested. She told me her skin even looked better—younger, fresher, and more glowing—and that she felt more centered and rejuvenated in everything she did.

In the two months that Krista experienced these changes, nothing else in her life was different other than the fact that she had adopted the Protocol. She didn't travel less—just on different days. She didn't start using an expensive new skin product or undergo a restrictive weight-loss program. Instead, she just finally synced with her body's seven-day schedule, and the transformation was profound.

That was more than four years ago. Today, Krista still follows the Protocol. She takes a break every now and then when her schedule gets too hectic, but otherwise, she says she couldn't imagine living her life out of rhythm anymore. While she had tried dozens of different diets, exercise routines, supplement plans, and other health trends in the past, she says only the Protocol has allowed her to fully reclaim her health, energy, and vitality.

Using the Protocol to Heal Your Body, Mind, and Spirit

The Protocol is a day-by-day plan that helps you sync your diet, exercise, and other lifestyle habits, along with any medical or self-care treatments you receive, with your body's seven-day inflammation-detoxification cycle in order to increase energy, prevent or reverse illness, and boost your overall health and well-being. Since I developed the Protocol over a decade ago, I've prescribed the plan to hundreds of patients—every single person I've treated—most of whom have benefited in incredible ways, as we'll detail throughout this book.

Because we all have the same seven-day cycle of inflammation and detoxification, the basics of the Protocol are universal and apply to everyone. But I still work closely with each and every patient to personalize the Protocol to better address their unique physical and emotional needs. I do this by gleaning as much information as I can about their illness or ailments so we make sure we target and treat these physical issues. I also spend time talking with them about their individual pain points, which are the emotional traumas or negative emotions and thoughts that may be making them sick. I do this in part by asking them the questions listed here, as well as by leading them through the other exercises and activities you'll find in chapter 5 to help identify emotional trauma.

Before we detail the Protocol's physical steps, I want you to consider the following questions, which should provide clues about what emotionally may be standing in your way of optimal physical health:

- Do you feel liberated in your body or life? Or do you feel stuck? If you feel stuck, what areas are making you feel that way?
- Do you feel like you're ever limiting yourself? If so, in which ways? Or do you feel like an external source is limiting you? If so, what is it?
- How does it feel to be you and live in your body every day?
- If you had to locate a physical part of your body where most of your emotional pain lives, where would that place be?
- If you had to create a name to call your emotional pain, what would it be?
- If you had to assign a color to your emotional pain, what color would it be?
- What times of the day does your body feel the best? What times of the day does your body feel the worst?
- Which activities do you wish you could do but feel like you can't, based on how you feel?
- Can you picture yourself being free of physical illness? If so, what are you doing? What does Healthy You look like?

These questions are designed to help you identify the source of the underlying issues that may be causing you to feel unwell. Giving your emotional trauma a location, a color, and a name helps create a strong visual, allowing you to better see and recognize the pain, which can help disarm it and make it feel less overwhelming. It may be helpful to write down your answers and refer back to them as you move through the book.

No matter what physical ailments and emotional trauma are at work, the next step I take with my patients is to teach them how to start using targeted nutrition on the Protocol to lower inflammation and speed the detoxification process. There are two ways to do this: by eating certain foods and by taking certain dietary supplements at specific times. Both the foods we eat and the dietary supplements we take provide nutrition that can help reduce your inflammatory load; better support the liver, kidneys, and lymphatic system; and increase the Cleanse, helping you eliminate more toxins, viral debris, and physical and emotional problems.

Educating yourself on the healing power of foods and dietary supplements and shifting your overall nutritional habits on a daily basis to better support your body's biorhythms take time and effort. But the investment is critical. Today, so many of us are removed from our nutrition, eating only what tastes good or is convenient without preparing our own meals or making conscientious decisions about what will best support our bodies. Similarly, plenty of people take supplements, but they don't know what these nutrients actually do in their bodies or how to time them to help the body heal. As I've seen in many of my patients, most people aren't getting the necessary nutrition they need to sustain life. And when the body's cells chronically fail to receive the nutrients they need, inflammation increases, digestion slows, and the body is forced to adopt new, unhealthy patterns to find what's missing. For these reasons, proper nutrition is critical on the Protocol. Let's take a look.

The Role of Food in the Protocol

The Protocol isn't a diet by any means. But what you eat and when you eat it can dramatically affect your body's seven-day cycle, either by supporting your body's circaseptan rhythms or working against them. On the Protocol, you have the chance to use food in a way no other diet or health plan does, allowing you to feed your body exactly what it needs on the days you need it the most while minimizing certain foods during the times when they'll do the most damage to your health and energy. This way, there's purpose and strategy in what you eat, and you're not just consuming healthy foods or avoiding allegedly unhealthy items at random: You power your body with the fuel it needs at the times it needs it for optimal healing, health, and performance.

More specifically, when you adopt the Protocol, you prioritize foods that support what's happening biologically in your body every day of your seven-day cycle. This means you give your body the nutrition it needs on Day One to recover, what it needs on Day Two to reset its inflammation baseline, what it needs on Day Three to restock your blood, and so on. Equally important, you minimize foods that increase inflammation—what are known as proinflammatory foods—along with those that can interfere with the function of your kidneys, liver, and lymphatic system on the days when they're all working overtime to detoxify. The more proinflammatory foods that you consume during the Cleanse, the more your body will hold onto inflammation, viral debris, illness, and old emotional trauma and prevent it from purging the chronic inflammation that causes disease.

On the Protocol, I don't want you to cut carbs, count calories, drink only shakes, or eat foods that taste like cardboard. The specific foods in the Protocol are all delicious, especially if you take the time to buy fresh fruits and veggies and prepare them at home—and with so many healthy recipe blogs and sites online, that's fairly easy to do. What's more, you can easily fit the foods of the Protocol into any diet you may already follow, whether you're keto, Paleo, gluten-free, et cetera.

When I talk about food throughout the book, you'll notice that I use the words *prioritize* and *minimize* instead of *eat* and *avoid*. That's because making major changes to your diet is difficult, and I want you to strive for good, not perfect. You might eat a food on a day when you're not supposed to, and that's okay. What's more important is that you try your best to prioritize and minimize certain foods as many days as possible. Don't stress about what you eat—anxiety doesn't improve health—but try instead to make conscientious choices about what you put in your mouth every day.

There's nothing you can't do for seven days. One week isn't a long time to commit to anything in the grand scheme of things, when you've already lived thousands of weeks of life. This is an opportunity to take one week to live mindfully, finding and feeling something new in your body every day for seven days. You can do this—I know it. Think of aligning your diet with your seven-day cycle as an unprecedented chance to hit the reset button and sync with your biorhythms to reconnect with your body in a way you never have before. When you start paying attention to what you eat, prioritizing foods that nourish the body's own rhythms and minimizing those that interfere with your cycle, you give your body a chance to do its thing without your interference. Committing to this intention for at least one week and being accountable to your goal are how you take back control of your body, energy, and overall well-being.

Healthy Foods to Prioritize on the Protocol

- **Seafood:** Fish and shellfish are high in omega-3 fat—one of the most anti-inflammatory nutrients you can consume. Seafood is also packed with protein, which will help your body better rebuild tissue and heal. Just be sure to choose types of fish that are low in mercury, PCBs, and other toxins. To find out the healthiest fish to eat, visit the Environmental Defense Fund's Seafood Selector at seafood.edf.org/guide /best.

- **Avocado:** I believe avocados are nature's perfect food. They contain a unique combination of monounsaturated, polyunsaturated, and saturated fats that is more similar to breast milk than any other food,[1] making avocados an ideal transitional food for newborns.[2] The creamy fruit is also high in energy and easy to digest, yet low in sugar, so it can help your body recover and refuel without adding the duress of digestion or too much sugar to your system. Avocados also contain more of certain types of antioxidants than any other food, including lutein, zeaxanthin, and glutathione, which work together to counter free radicals, or harmful molecules that can damage cells and cause disease.[3]

- **Citrus fruits:** Any kind of fresh, whole fruit is great to prioritize on the Protocol: Fruit is rich in vitamins, minerals, fiber, antioxidants, and phytochemicals (healthy plant compounds), all of which can help drive down inflammation, boost energy, and help the body heal. But citrus fruits in particular, including oranges, grapefruits, limes, and lemons, are especially beneficial for your seven-day cycle because they help improve immune function, lower inflammation, and speed detoxification. Citrus fruits contain concentrated amounts of immune-boosting vitamin C, along with citrus flavonoids, which have been shown by studies to fight free radicals, decreasing inflammation.[4] Citrus flavonoids also have strong antiviral effects, helping thwart all kinds of infections, from the common cold to Epstein-Barr,[5] while studies show consuming more citrus may reduce cancer risk by as much as 10 percent in the instance of breast cancer.[6] Citrus fruits also play a strong role in detoxication, helping the liver produce enzymes that flush toxins[7] while safeguarding liver cells from harm.[8]

- **Dark leafy greens:** You likely already know that dark, leafy greens are nutritional powerhouses—they're low in calories and carbohydrates but packed with an array of vitamins, minerals, antioxidants, and phytochemicals that are not found in many other foods. Leafy greens like kale, spinach, collards, broccoli, bok choy, mustard greens, arugula, and beet greens have all been shown by research to drive down inflammation in remarkable and significant ways.[9] Many also contain the nutrient quercetin, which research shows can lower inflammation as effectively as aspirin or ibuprofen.[10] Additionally, dark leafy greens contain high amounts of the plant pigment chlorophyll, which studies show can act as a strong detoxicant in the body, helping to eliminate toxins, including those that may be carcinogenic.[11]

- **Nuts:** When you get on the Protocol, you'll want to minimize foods high in sugar and/or refined carbs, including potato chips, crackers, granola bars, breakfast cereal, cookies, and other processed foods, all of which can increase inflammation. But it's easier to cut this junk from your daily diet when you have nuts in your nutritional arsenal. Not only do nuts provide the same satisfying, salty crunch that many processed snacks do but they're also high in anti-inflammatory antioxidants *and* anti-inflammatory fats[12]—a combination not found in many other foods. That's one reason why a group of scientists ranked almonds in particular as the number-one healthiest food out of one thousand possible foods.[13] In addition to almonds, look for walnuts, pecans, and other tree nuts, but try to minimize peanuts. Peanuts, which are technically a legume, not a nut, contain a type of mold called aflatoxin, a known carcinogen that increases inflammation, according to research.[14]

- **Beans and lentils:** The reason I like beans and lentils for patients on the Protocol is because they're a more nutritious, more filling substitute for many proinflammatory, refined starches on store shelves. Packed with protein, fiber, and complex carbs, beans and lentils don't spike blood sugar like refined breads, pastas, and other simple carbs do. Instead, they provide consistent energy, helping your body refuel, recover, and rebuild. Beans and lentils are a surprising source of anti-inflammatory antioxidants. In fact, small red beans contain more antioxidants than wild or cultivated blueberries,[15] according to research, while black beans boast ten times the antioxidants found in most fruit.[16]

- **Coconut and avocado oil:** Most foods, whether you pick them up at the store or order them from a restaurant, are made with chemically extracted vegetable oils like soybean, corn, sunflower, peanut, and cottonseed. While cheap to produce, these refined oils are high in omega-6 fat, which boosts inflammation, especially in the amounts most Americans consume.[17] These oils also oxidize or spoil easily, which produces compounds toxic to human health.[18] Some vegetable oils have also been linked to liver damage,[19] which will interfere with your body's ability to detoxify.

  For these reasons, I recommend swapping the cooking oils in your kitchen for coconut and/or avocado oil. I like coconut oil because, unlike most other oils, it's processed directly by your liver, where it's converted into energy immediately rather than being stored as fat.[20] The neutral-tasting oil also acts as a detoxicant[21] and is one of few cooking oils that won't oxidize, or go rancid. On the other hand, avocado oil, which has a slightly buttery, grassy flavor, can increase your absorption of nutrients from other foods[22] and has been shown by research to be an effective anti-inflammatory—so much so that the oil is used clinically in parts of Europe to help treat arthritis.[23] You can also use olive oil in cold dressings, but I don't recommend cooking with it, since it has a lower smoke point and can turn carcinogenic at high heat.

- **Honey:** Sugar is one of the most proinflammatory foods you can eat, which is why I suggest you minimize it as much as possible on the Protocol. But that doesn't mean you have to give up on all things sweet. Honey in moderation is a great sugar substitute for coffee and tea or drizzled over whole-grain toast, plain oatmeal, or in goat's milk yogurt. Honey is all-natural (compared to refined cane sugar, corn syrup, dextrose, and other processed sweeteners) and low on the glycemic index, meaning it won't spike your blood sugar and consequently stress out your body.[24] Honey also acts as an antiviral, antimicrobial, and anti-inflammatory to boot, all of which can help safeguard your body through your seven-day cycle.

- **Stevia:** This all-natural sugar substitute, made from the leaves of the South American stevia plant, is one hundred to three hundred times sweeter than table sugar but without the commensurate calories and blood sugar spike found in sugar-derived sweeteners. Stevia also doesn't have any of the chemicals or other harmful additives that sucralose (Splenda), aspartame (Equal), and other noncaloric sugar substitutes do. Unlike these toxic sweeteners, stevia can actually help regulate your blood sugar levels,[25] has strong antiviral effects,[26] and is even used by some to help treat Lyme disease.[27] Available in liquid and powder form, stevia can be used anywhere you'd use regular sugar, including in coffee, tea, oatmeal, yogurt, and cooking and baking.

Unhealthy Foods to Minimize on the Protocol

- **Sugar and refined carbs:** Added sugar is one of the most inflammatory nutrients you can consume, despite its prevalence in three-quarters of all our packaged foods and almost everything else we eat.[28] Described as a "poison" and "toxin" by top scientists,[29] added sugar instantly drives up inflammation and can damage your liver as much as alcohol does, according to research.[30] Sugar, even when consumed in allegedly "healthy" items like sports drinks, smoothies, protein bars, granola, and some gluten- or grain-free snacks, can also increase appetite, limit nutrient absorption,[31] cause weight gain and mood swings, and prevent the body from properly detoxifying.[32]

It's not just added sugar you have to watch out for, either. Refined carbs, including white bread, white pasta, white rice, many breakfast cereals, potato and vegetable chips, cookies, crackers, and similar packaged snack and meal foods, are processed grains that have been stripped of their fiber, bran, and other healthful nutrients, causing them to break down into simple sugar and trigger the same harmful effects in the body. Most refined carbs contain a lot of calories but almost no nutrition, in addition to unhealthy vegetable oils and chemical preservatives, emulsifiers, dyes, and other additives that can increase inflammation and interfere with the body's ability to function optimally.

Minimizing added sugars and refined carbs isn't easy, since both are in the majority of foods found in supermarkets, restaurants, and take-out items. What I suggest you do instead is try to prioritize whole foods that look like they came directly from a farm, not a factory—items like whole fruits, whole vegetables, dry or canned beans, dry or canned lentils, and nuts. You can also add some whole grains to your diet like quinoa, farro, brown rice, and 100 percent whole-grain bread and pasta, but be sure to read labels to make sure these products are made with 100 percent whole grains and don't contain added sugar or other toxic ingredients.

- **Red meat:** Red meat, especially cuts that are high in fat, can be detrimental to your body's seven-day cycle, driving up inflammation and interfering with your liver's detoxification activity. Red meat is a double whammy for your liver because it has to process protein and fat at the same time, which is a stressful process when you do it on a daily basis.[33] Red meat contains high amounts of a sugar molecule known as Neu5Gc, which research shows can cause an immune response in the body that increases cancer risk and fuels tumor growth.[34] Industrially raised beef is also full of hormones, steroids, and stress-related toxins produced by animals that are fed an unnatural diet and quartered and slaughtered in traumatic conditions. If you don't want to give up red meat, try to prioritize grass-fed cuts that are lower in fat like bison, venison, and 96 percent lean hamburger or steak, and limit your intake to once or twice weekly.

- **Cow's dairy:** Despite the fact that milk, yogurt, cheese, and ice cream are everywhere, 65 percent of people can't digest the sugar found in milk, meaning they're lactose intolerant.[35] In addition, some people have an outright sensitivity or allergy to whey and casein, the two proteins found in cow's dairy, which causes an immune reaction that's separate from lactose intolerance. Both can hinder your body's ability to heal and detoxify, which is why I recommend everyone on the Protocol minimize cow's dairy and foods that contain whey and casein. If you want a dairy substitute, look for products made from goat's milk, which contains less lactose than cow's milk, with smaller fat globules, making it easier to digest.[36] Goat's dairy also has a different type of casein—A2 beta casein compared to A1 beta casein found in most conventional cow's dairy—which doesn't trigger the same allergic response and inflammation.[37] Finally, because of its biological makeup, goat's dairy doesn't need to be homogenized like cow's dairy does, obviating the process, which produces harmful free radicals.[38]

- **Nightshade vegetables:** Nightshade vegetables like eggplants, white potatoes (but not sweet potatoes or yams), tomatoes, bell peppers, cayenne pepper, and paprika contain a toxin called solanine, which is fatal to humans in concentrated amounts. In smaller quantities, solanine can irritate your gastrointestinal tract and cause inflammation. Some people are also sensitive or allergic to nightshades, which can trigger an autoimmune response by the body that can also cause chronic and systemic levels of inflammation.[39]

- **Corn:** Whether you realize it or not, corn is ubiquitous in the foods we eat, found in almost everything as cornstarch, corn syrup, corn oil, corn flour, or corn feed, which is given to most of the animals we eat.[40] The problem with all this corn is that it's high in cellulose, a tough insoluble fiber that humans can't digest,[41] causing your body to work overtime. Corn also contains a lot of sugar, spiking your blood sugar levels and ratcheting up inflammation. More than 90 percent of all corn is also genetically modified (GM).[42] While big agricultural companies might lead you to believe that GM crops are no big deal, independent studies show eating too much GM foods can have a toxic effect, especially on the liver.[43]

The Role of Supplements in the Protocol

Just like the foods you eat, dietary supplements are a big part of the Protocol, since what you consume, whether it's a food, drink, or a concentrated supplement, will either support your body's seven-day cycle or work against it. Similar to eating certain foods, when you prioritize taking targeted supplements on certain days, you nourish everything good going on in your body while increasing your ability to fight inflammation and detoxify. Taken at the right times as part of the Protocol, supplements can increase energy, treat or reverse disease, boost weight loss, improve how you look and feel, and bolster your overall health and well-being.

If you've taken supplements in the past without any measurable results, I would encourage you to rethink any preconceived notions or disappointment you may have around them. First, I'm betting you didn't take the types of supplements I'm about to recommend, most of which come directly from plants. Studies show that plant-based supplements like dandelion root, turmeric, and milk thistle can be as powerful as prescription drugs, many of which are also made from plants.[44]

The supplements I recommend on the Protocol that aren't plant based don't come from a lab but from the natural world. Royal jelly, for example, is produced by honeybees, probiotics are live strains of bacteria, and vitamin B_{12}—a common deficiency affecting at least 40 percent of all Americans, according to studies[45]—is derived from animal sources.

On the Protocol, *when* you take a supplement is equally as important as *what* you actually take. When you consume certain nutrients at certain times, supplements will work far more effectively because they will correspond with or complement what's happening in your body. For example, taking activated charcoal and dandelion root helps trap toxins and stimulates the liver to get rid of excess toxins, respectively. Taking these supplements Days Six and Seven when you know your body is detoxifying will help you eliminate more inflammatory chemicals and other harmful substances.

Taking probiotics Days One through Five, on the other hand, will help restore levels of healthy bacteria in your microbiome—the body's community of microorganisms that are critical to overall health and mood—while also helping you regrow a more nourishing gut lining, which the body sheds every seven days. But you don't need or want to take probiotics on Days Six and Seven, when your body is busy shedding your gut lining, as that's literally money down the toilet.

In total, I recommend everyone take eight supplements in order to get the best possible results from the Protocol. You don't have to take all or even any of them for the program to work—syncing your diet, exercise, and lifestyle habits with your circaseptan rhythms will help you fight disease and boost your overall physical, mental, and spiritual wellness. But adding these supplements on the days recommended can *significantly* boost your body's ability to grow, rebuild, fight inflammation, detoxify, and heal, according to your seven-day cycle.

I know supplements can be pricey. If cost is an issue, compare products online and look for companies that offer subscription deals at reduced rates. Be sure to pick supplements with the NSF International seal, which ensures the product contains what it says it does without any potentially toxic ingredients or unidentified fillers. Without this seal, there's no guarantee you're getting a product that contains the nutrient you want, which means you could be throwing away your money. When possible, also be sure to choose liquid supplements, which are much more absorbable than tablets, pills, or powders.

You can think of adopting the Protocol without supplements like keeping an orchid in your house in any room you want—it'll do just fine if you tend to it. But if you keep that orchid in a room with an ideal amount of humidity and sunlight while giving it just as much water and fertilizer as it needs at exactly the right times, your orchid will flourish and flower beautifully. The same is true of your body when you follow the Protocol with supplements.

On the Protocol, you'll take five supplements on Days One through Five and three supplements on Days Six and Seven. While this daily schedule matters immensely, what doesn't is what time you take them each day. I recommend supplementing in the morning because that's when your body best metabolizes nutrients, but if the only time you can remember to take your supplements is at night, that's when you should do so. It's like exercise—for some people, it's easier to work out in the morning while others prefer to work out at night. What matters the most, however, is that you do it.

To help you remember to take your supplements, I suggest developing a ritual around them in which you look at taking these nutrients as a prime window of wellness. Don't just swallow blindly but do so with purpose, repeating the day's daily mantra beforehand and visualizing the nutrients healing your body (FYI, you'll find a daily mantra and supplement visualization for each day of the week in chapters 7 through 13). You can also add other ritualistic elements to your supplement taking, whether you want to thank the supplements for doing their job before you take them or practice deep breathing afterward. Creating a ritual not only helps make supplements a habit but also increases the efficacy of the nutrients: When you believe something will work and visualize its healing effects in your body, it has a much greater chance of improving your wellness, according to a body of research.

Four Things to Know about Dietary Supplements

1. **Talk before you take.** Always consult your doctor or other health care provider before taking a new supplement. Some supplements can interact with prescription medications or negatively affect existing medical conditions. Being open and honest with your doctor can also help him or her better heal you.
2. **Follow instructions.** For each supplement listed here, follow product instructions for dosing or talk with your health care provider about what dose is best for you.
3. **Look for liquid.** Liquid supplements are more absorbable than tab-

lets, pills, or powders, since your body doesn't have to break anything down to get at the good stuff. To find liquid supplements, look online or ask at your local health-food store.

4. **Think quality before economy.** I know supplements are a financial investment. But if you're going to spend any money, I suggest finding high-quality brands—it might cost you a few extra bucks, but it's better to spend more to get a product you know is potent than saving several dollars to get something that won't work. To find a high-quality brand, do some online research and look for products certified with the NSF International seal, which guarantees a supplement contains what it claims it does.

Supplements to Help Heal and Rebuild (Days One through Five)

- **Turmeric:** There's a reason turmeric has been called "the most effective supplement in existence."[46] The spice, which gives curry its yellow color, contains the compound curcumin, which studies show can lower inflammation levels and decrease pain as effectively as ibuprofen (Advil) without any side effects.[47] The compound also fights inflammation on a molecular level, proving to be more beneficial than many other anti-inflammatory supplements and drugs.[48] Curcumin has also been shown to increase production of brain-derived neurotrophic factor, a hormone that helps build new neurons, boosting cognitive function and limiting depression and dementia.[49] What's more, studies show curcumin can help prevent heart disease,[50] ward off and even kill cancer cells,[51] and fight a number of other chronic illnesses and diseases. Why not take curcumin instead of turmeric? Research shows that other compounds in turmeric, which is the whole plant, make it more effective than the isolated compound curcumin alone.[52]

  Pro tip: I suggest swallowing turmeric thirty minutes before or after the other supplements for Days One through Five, since turmeric can block the absorption of other nutrients. Additionally, the powers of turmeric are best unlocked when combined with black pepper, so look for a brand that contains BioPerine, the trade name for black pepper extract, which increases the bioavailability of curcumin by 2,000 percent.[53] You may already be cooking with turmeric, which is great, but you do need to take it in supplement form to reap the full benefits: while curcumin is the active compound in turmeric, the spice contains only about 3 percent curcumin, making it difficult to consume enough to fully enjoy its anti-inflammatory properties.[54]

- **Wheatgrass:** You've likely seen shoppers in health-food stores chugging shots of bright-green wheatgrass. As it turns out, there's a very good reason this "hippie drink" has a cult following. Sold as a juice, powder, and supplement, wheatgrass is made from the leaves of the wheat plant (note: it doesn't contain gluten) and is loaded with vitamins, antioxidants, and seventeen different amino acids, including the nine essential amino acids the body needs to build muscle and sustain immune function. More impressively, wheatgrass is one of the best dietary sources of the green-plant pigment chlorophyll, a powerful anti-inflammatory[55] that also helps the liver get rid of toxins.[56] Known to stimulate weight loss, wheatgrass has also been shown to kill cancer cells with rates up to 65 percent.[57]

  Pro tip: The best way to ingest wheatgrass is as a liquid, but you don't need to go to a health-food store every day to get your daily dose: You can make the drink at home by mixing a high-quality powder with water. To find a high-quality powder, look for a certification or seal from NSF International, which tests supplements for efficacy and purity.

- **Probiotics:** You likely already know that probiotics are live microorganisms that help us digest and process food. But did you know that they can also work wonders in improving your mood? That may sound a little woo-woo, but it's science: Probiotics support the community of bacteria in the gut's microbiome, where we produce most of the feel-good hormone serotonin needed for mood stability. A healthy gut-brain connection can prevent anxiety and depression[58] and allow you to heal from trauma more easily. What's more, probiotics are imperative for immune function and digestive health—one reason why my patients who take probiotics on the Protocol have experienced up to 35 percent more weight loss than when they tried to lose weight without probiotics and the Protocol.

Pro tip: Probiotics are live organisms, so any supplement you choose should have an expiration date. Be sure to confirm that whatever you buy isn't past its prime. While consistency and remembering to take your supplements every day is the most important piece of the puzzle, popping a probiotic on an empty stomach will help your body best absorb the microorganisms.[59] This way, you'll have less stomach acid, which can kill live healthy bacteria.

- **Royal jelly:** Royal jelly is one of the most unique substances on the planet. This sticky material is produced by worker bees to feed queen bees, helping them live longer—one reason why numerous studies show this nutrient-rich jelly can prevent aging in people, too.[60] Packed with a rare combo of fatty acids, essential B vitamins, amino acids, antioxidants, and other nutrients, royal jelly can help reduce inflammation in immune cells,[61] increase collagen production,[62] and help tissue heal faster.[63]

  Pro tip: No need to look for royal jelly as a liquid: Purchase the substance in its natural gelatinous form and put the recommended dose under your tongue.

- **Lemon balm:** Used as a digestive tonic for centuries in the Middle East, this herb has strong antiviral effects,[64] helping protect the body from illness and infection. Studies show that lemon balm can also lower inflammation[65] and increase thyroid regulation.[66] The herb, which belongs to the mint family, also boosts cognitive function,[67] according to studies, so much so that lemon balm has been used to help treat those with anxiety and Alzheimer's disease.[68]

Pro tip: It's easy to find liquid lemon balm in tincture form, which you can mix into water or juice.

Supplements to Help Detoxify (Days Six and Seven)

- **Milk thistle extract:** Few supplements actually protect the liver, which is what your body desperately needs Days Six and Seven when this organ is working overtime to clear inflammation and other toxins from the body. That's why milk thistle extract is amazing: This inexpensive supplement has been shown to prevent toxins from attaching to liver cells,[69] so much so that the extract has been used to treat people with acute liver conditions like cirrhosis, fatty liver disease, and liver cancer. Milk thistle is also a potent anti-inflammatory, capable of reducing oxidative damage in the brain,[70] and has been shown to lower blood sugar[71] and even kill cancer cells.[72]

  Pro tip: Those with allergies to ragweed or other plants from the same family should avoid taking milk thistle and can supplement with ginseng instead.[73]

- **Dandelion root:** Similar to milk thistle, dandelion root also protects the liver from toxins and oxidative stress,[74] in part due to the plant's impressive antioxidant levels. The root has a strong anti-inflammatory effect,[75] helping to reduce the number of inflammatory markers in the body's cells on Days Six and Seven. Dandelion has also been shown to prevent viruses[76] and harmful bacteria[77] from replicating, which is exactly what you want and need on Days Six and Seven. Dandelion is also a diuretic and mild laxative, helping stimulate the body to excrete toxins.

  Pro tip: Like milk thistle, anyone with allergies to ragweed and plants part of the same family should not supplement with dandelion root. Take ginseng instead.

- **Activated charcoal:** Activated charcoal has become increasingly trendy in recent years, showing up in soaps, toothpastes, shampoos, and other personal-care products, as more people realize the nutrient's incredible potential. Activated charcoal is nontoxic, especially porous, and negatively charged, enabling it to attract toxins and trap them before your body absorbs them—why it's been used for years in medical clinics and hospitals to help treat poisoning.[78] Activated charcoal's ability to bind toxins is no joke: Studies show the supplement can reduce our absorption of a harmful substance by up to 74 percent.[79] This makes the supplement extremely advantageous on Days Six and Seven, when high levels of toxins are circulating through our cells and bloodstream.

Pro tip: Since activated charcoal can reduce the body's ability to absorb chemicals, including those in prescription medications, be sure to talk to your doctor before adding to your regimen if you're already taking prescription drugs.

Supplements to Support Specific Issues

In addition to the general Protocol, there are specific ailments that I see a lot that the plan can help the body heal from. Here, I'll share information about several specific supplements for those dealing with thyroid issues, menopause or perimenopause, anxiety and/or depression, and viral infections. If you have any of these conditions, adding some specific nutrients to your supplement regimen on Days One through Five can help ease and even reverse symptoms while helping your body better rebuild and heal. Again, be sure to consult your doctor before you begin taking any of the following supplements.

Thyroid Issues (Days One through Five)

- **Vitamin B_{12}:** Millions of Americans are deficient in vitamin B_{12}, with conservative estimates that up to 15 percent of the general population is short on the essential nutrient.[80] This is a big problem, especially if you have a sluggish thyroid, or hypothyroidism—a condition researchers say may be caused and aggravated by low B_{12} levels.[81] Taking a supplement can help ease symptoms and even treat low thyroid function.[82]

- **Cat's claw:** More and more research shows that viruses, like Epstein-Barr, may contribute to thyroid disorders.[83] That's where cat's claw comes into play. This supplement, made from tropical vines that grow in Central and South America, acts as an antiviral agent, helping to limit the spread of and treat viruses in the body, sometimes even more effectively than antiviral drugs, according to studies.[84]

- **Methylfolate:** You're probably already familiar with the essential B vitamin folate—methylfolate is just one form of folate. Taking methylfolate can help people with thyroid problems who also have a mutation of a gene known as MTHFR, or methylenetetrahydrofolate reductase. Common mutations of the gene can lead to high levels of an amino acid known as homocysteine and low levels of folate. Supplementing with methylfolate can help ease and even reverse symptoms brought on by excess homocysteine and low folate.

Menopause and Perimenopause (Days One through Five)

- **Red raspberry leaf extract:** The leaves of the delicious berry by the same name have been used for years to help ease morning sickness for pregnant women.[85] Known as a "uterine tonic," red raspberry leaf also helps reduce PMS symptoms, cramping, hot flashes, and nausea.

- **Methylfolate:** Studies show that supplementing with folate may reduce hot flashes by up to 57 percent.[86] Methylfolate is the most bioavailable form of folate, meaning your body has the easiest time absorbing and incorporating the nutrient.

Anxiety and/or Depression (Days One through Five)

- **Vitamin B$_{12}$:** Reams of research show vitamin B$_{12}$ is critical to good mood, whether you're suffering from clinical anxiety or depression, or simply want to feel more optimistic and joyful on a regular basis. This essential B vitamin helps produce the feel-good hormone serotonin, which is why some doctors now treat depression and other mood disorders with B_{12} supplements.[87]

Viral Infections (Days One through Five)

- **Lysine:** One of nine essential amino acids, lysine has impressive research to show it can help fight viral infections, including everything from cold sores[88] to shingles, mononucleosis, and Epstein-Barr.

- **Cat's claw:** Cat's claw can help fight viral infections[89] and ease symptoms, according to multiple studies, sometimes even more effectively than prescription drugs.[90] The Amazonian plant contains several unique compounds that act as powerful anti-inflammatories[91] and is being studied for use in helping to treat arthritis and even Alzheimer's.[92]

THE EMOTIONAL PART
OF THE PROTOCOL

CHAPTER 5

P alm Springs is literally a hotbed of secrets. The sweltering desert hide-away, less than two hours by car and only a forty-five-minute flight from Los Angeles, is where John F. Kennedy allegedly began his affair with Marilyn Monroe and where mobsters like Al Capone kept hideouts in old hot springs. Many celebrities have or had second homes there, including Frank Sina-tra, Leonardo DiCaprio, Liberace, Elvis Presley, and the Kardashians, and like many vacation homes, nearly all have their own mysteries and memories for any who've visited or lived inside.

I knew plenty about Palm Springs before I met TJ, but I became much more familiar with the "playground of the stars," as the Californian city is called, when we started working together several years ago. The superstar actor had spent his childhood there, where his father, who was an even more famous actor than his son, had once owned a palatial palm-edged estate named Foxtail. The home, named after a variety of palm tree that dominates the desert, was a massive estate, with several swimming pools, tennis courts, and a handful of casitas on acres of meticulously manicured lawns. I'm not quite sure how much TJ ever looked back on his early years at Foxtail, but when we started working together, we realized that what had happened there when the actor was only nine had upended his health and happiness for years to come.

At first recall, TJ's primary memory of the estate may not seem significant. He and his brother, Geoff, had gotten ahold of one of their father's go-karts and were racing the car around the estate when something went wrong—not an uncommon occurrence when you mix kids with motorized machines—and the brothers crashed the go-kart into a palm tree. The steering wheel jammed into TJ's stomach, and the expensive go-kart was destroyed.

At the time, TJ was terrified to tell his father. While no one had been seri-ously injured, the paparazzi continually outside the fences hadn't seen the acci-dent, and his father had enough money to buy the go-kart manufacturer, not to mention a new car, TJ's father had a long history of angry outbursts, including many that were caught on camera. And this time, he was outraged, yelling at both boys for hours while telling TJ in particular how worthless he was. The actor told me it's the first time he ever remembers feeling shame, humiliation, and disgrace.

One month after the accident, TJ developed a peculiar problem: He stopped sweating properly. He could still perspire, but only in small amounts, which quickly became a problem in the searing California heat. Several months later, the boy began breaking out in a bright-red rash all over his stomach and legs, so richly colored and extensive that, at times, it looked like a giant birthmark over his lower body. The rash didn't itch, but it could be painful—and it was always embarrassing.

TJ's mother quickly sent him to dozens of different doctors, none of whom could figure out what was causing the rash or his sweating malfunction. Year after year, the actor's rash and perspiration problems persisted, until he stopped wearing shorts altogether. He became so self-conscious of his body, despite his growing success in films and TV, he began to feel uncomfortable doing anything active or outside.

When I first met TJ, he was in his late fifties and had seen nearly a hundred different doctors and other health care providers for his condition but still didn't have any answers. He asked if I could help him, and at first, I was admittedly unsure what I would be able to contribute. But I was willing to try; I already knew and had seen what the Protocol had done for dozens of my other celebrity clients.

My first question to TJ is probably one you can guess by now: He was born on a Friday. When I explained the Protocol, he told me he was intrigued and wanted to test my "theory," pledging to get his blood drawn daily by the family's in-house doctor. One week later, he sent me the results, even though he didn't need me or any other medical professional to interpret what even he could see by himself in the numbers: His inflammatory levels spiked considerably on Friday. He was sold, and began making small changes to his daily schedule in order to line up with his body's seven-day inflammation-detoxification cycle.

I was proud of TJ, but for the actor and many of my other patients, adopting the Protocol is only the first step on the journey they have to take in order to heal their bodies and transform their lives. That's because you can eat all the right foods, take all the right supplements, and do all the right activities at the right times, but if you have major unresolved emotional trauma or persistent negative emotions or thoughts, you won't be able to fully heal from whatever ails you.

After speaking with TJ, I told him I believed that he must have experienced some emotional trauma shortly before he developed the sweating problems and rash. When I asked what he could remember around the time before he got sick, he immediately told me about the go-kart accident and the shame and humiliation he faced from his father.

Suddenly, it made sense to both of us: TJ's first feelings of shame and embarrassment had implanted in his body and eventually manifested as a physical form of shame and embarrassment in a very visible rash. In other words, TJ's emotional trauma had found a physical outlet in his body. As long as the actor didn't address the trauma or negative emotions provoked by the incident, his incessant sweating and rash would persist.

My work with TJ then shifted from helping him not only adopt the Protocol but also unpack the emotional baggage that was weighing him down. I'm not a therapist, nor do I pretend to be one, but I tried to help the actor see that his purpose, destiny, and identity were separate from his father's and that he didn't have to carry or absorb his father's anger. I suggested he start meditating and practice mindfulness, not only so he could try to forgive his father but also so he could learn to be more present in the moment, remaining in the here and now rather than staying stuck in his painful past.

Three months after TJ began addressing the trauma, along with the help of the Protocol, the rash he had lived with for almost fifty years started to recede. Six months later, the actor began to sweat normally for the first time since he was just nine years old. He was ecstatic.

In TJ's story, it was relatively easy to determine the emotional trauma behind his physical issues. But for the majority of my patients—and perhaps for you, too—identifying the trauma contributing to your fatigue, weight gain, chronic pain, illness, or disease isn't always easy. Sometimes it can take months or even years to figure out if a certain incident, relationship, or other part of your past is making you ill.

While it's helpful, you don't necessarily need to determine the exact trauma causing your illness in order to overcome the negative emotions and thought patterns associated with it. Instead, you can identify the negative emotions and thoughts and work toward creating positive, healthier ones in their place.

No matter what you do, it's really important to understand how negative emotions and thoughts can make you sick. While we covered some ways emotional trauma can trigger physical trauma in chapter 2 (see page 21), in short, negative emotions increase inflammation, which can persist for months or even years after you experience a trauma—why children who experience tragedies like rape or the death of a parent early in life are more prone to illness in adulthood, according to studies.[1]

You already know that humans store emotional trauma in our conscious and subconscious minds. But what most people don't realize is that we can also hold on to trauma in our cells, muscles, and other tissues. From a scientific standpoint, researchers believe that emotional trauma can shock the nervous system into a constant state of fight-or-flight, even if you no longer consciously think about the original incident.[2] On the other hand, when the body releases a trauma through physical, mental, or emotional intervention, the nervous system can relax and initiate a healing response. Studies show terminally ill cancer patients who suddenly go into remission often credit the release of emotional trauma as the reason for their unexpected healing.[3] Releasing emotional trauma has also been fingered by researchers as the reason why some people start crying or become emotional after deep-tissue massage or acupuncture, which can help the body excavate and release old emotions trapped in tissue.[4]

Every emotion and thought we feel and think also creates a cascade of chemicals or neurotransmitters in the brain that influences the health and activity of the body's cells.[5] Positive emotions and thoughts trigger positive cellular effects, while negative emotions and thoughts, especially those we feel and think over and over again, cause negative cellular effects.

Just because the body stores emotional trauma doesn't mean you're doomed to be a victim of your past. You can work through trauma, no matter how deep-seated, and create healthier, more positive emotions and thoughts to help heal yourself. The first step is to identify and acknowledge the trauma itself or the negative emotions and thoughts driving you to feel unwell. The second step is to work through this trauma or reverse negative emotions and thoughts by replacing them with positive ones.

I want to empower you to step into your own strength. Emotions and thoughts are extremely powerful in the body and our lives at large, and if you believe something with your body, mind, soul, and spirit, it can and will likely happen. Similarly, if you believe you can change how you feel and heal your body, you can. If you don't believe in your own strength and power to heal your body, you may stay stuck in a place of not feeling good or having suboptimal health for years.

Scientists already know that visualization—imagining what you want to happen—and belief are extremely powerful tools in medicine. Studies show that cancer patients who visualize healthy outcomes increase their immune function and overall well-being while helping reduce the severity of their symptoms.[6] Similarly, research has found that when a drug or treatment is *believed* to cure an ailment or reduce symptoms, it often achieves that effect, even if the drug is a sugar pill or the treatment is a sham.[7]

The common thread in all of this is empowerment through education. When you learn that a certain supplement can lower inflammation, for example, *and* you believe that nutrient will lower inflammation, you're more likely to achieve the result. Your mental and emotional buy-in triggers a mind-body integration that will help you trust, understand, and cross-promote the healing benefits of any drug, supplement, treatment, or everyday action. When you believe an intervention will work and have full faith in your body's overall ability to heal itself, you let go of a precognitive commitment of what your body or health has to be.

What it really comes down to is mind over matter. If you believe you're someone who will get sick, that's the body you'll walk around in. On the other hand, if you believe you're resilient and can overcome anything, you will. And when it comes to overcoming emotional trauma, you have to believe that your body wants to work with you rather than against you.

Identifying Emotional Trauma

The body handles emotional trauma the same way it does physical trauma. When the body experiences a physical trauma like an injury or infection, it creates inflammation in the area that's hurt or infected. When we experience an emotional trauma, the body creates inflammation in the physical part associated with that trauma. Emotional trauma doesn't have to be extreme, but can result from the loss of a beloved childhood pet, for example, or a bad experience at a first job, a definitive fight with a romantic partner, or a toxic teacher in grade school. And it doesn't need to manifest as a major illness like cancer or a full-body rash: Emotional trauma can also present as a minor ailment, like an achy knee, bad back, premature hair loss, or persistent headache. These are only instances, however, that point to the extraordinary connection between emotional trauma and illness. For example, almost every woman I know who's had breast cancer also has an emotional trauma or pain point in her mother-child relationship, whether that's an issue with her own mother or her identity as a mother. That's because mothers nurture their babies at their breasts, so any emotional trauma in the mother-child relationship will physically inflame the chest area. Similarly, the reason we get an upset stomach when we're anxious is because the stomach is the threshold of responsibility, so anything that makes us feel like we're forsaking or jeopardizing our responsibilities can make us sick to our stomach, literally. After women experience sexual trauma, it often shows up physically as cervical dysplasia or cancer or ovarian cancer.

Let's go back to Katie, whose story I shared in chapter 2. Katie had breast cancer, which to me indicates an unhealthy mother-child relationship. Knowing this, I asked Katie to think about whether she was feeling a lot of grief and, if so, what might be causing this anguish. I also asked her how she felt about her mother as well as herself as a mother.

As it turns out, Katie was never close with her mother, who was jealous of her. Katie has always been well-liked and beautiful, both on the inside and out, and growing up, her mother resented the attention her daughter received. Katie told me that her mother often shunned her, which caused her to feel bad about herself and unhappy in her relationship with her mother. This anguish took seat in Katie's chest, particularly in her breast, which is where mothers first connect with their daughters and sons. Flash forward, and that anguish years later turned into breast cancer, which now threatened to take Katie's life. In order to help her heal, I first had to help Katie let go of the grief she had kept for so long there.

While you don't need to identify the particular emotional trauma that may be causing you to physically feel unwell, doing so will help you heal more quickly and effectively on the Protocol. But how do you begin to assess your personal emotional trauma? Here are three quick exercises to help you, along with a longer activity to help you pinpoint the negative emotions or thoughts affecting you, based on the physical area of your body where you feel unwell.

First, take the time to think about your most agonizing memory and who or what made the experience so painful. Typically, our most difficult emotional experience is the one driving our bodies' bus, so to speak, physically, mentally, and emotionally. While this can be painful, your answers will provide insight into what may be haunting your health and preventing you from feeling well.

Next, think back to the time in your life when you last felt physically well. What happened around this time that may have triggered your condition? Consider specific incidents or events, as well as how your relationships with others may have changed.

Now, find a quiet place where you can be alone. Sit with your eyes closed and try to quiet your mind and energy. When you feel calm, think about where on your body you feel the most emotional—not physical—pain, and point to that spot. Ask yourself how this area of emotional hurt makes you feel, using as many adjectives as you can to describe your feelings, whether you feel fearful, heartbroken, or abandoned, until you're out of words. Give this emotional hurt a name, which will become apparent to you as you uncover the truth, and a color to help you visualize it. Giving your emotional pain a location, name, and color helps create a strong visual, allowing you to better see and recognize the pain, which can help disarm it and make it feel less overwhelming.

Finally, the following activity with prompts can help you determine which negative emotions and thoughts are causing you to feel unwell. The activity is inspired in part by best-selling author Louise Hay, who was one of the most influential healers of our time. Like me, Hay believed that every physical condition is caused by a specific emotion, set of emotions, or thought patterns associated with the area of your body where you feel unwell. In the following activity, I've combined Hay's philosophy with my own to help you determine the negative emotions and thought patterns that may be driving your physical illness or issues, based on where in your body you're experiencing symptoms. Then, in the subsequent section, I'll show you how to heal these negative emotions and thought patterns using a similar exercise.

Exercise: How to Identify Emotional Trauma

To complete the following activity, carefully consider your answers to the three questions that pertain to any area of your body where you feel unwell. As you do so, write down whatever words, insights, or memories come to mind without analyzing or judging them. If you find yourself stuck on a particular question, come back to it when you feel ready or when you have more mental clarity.

Remember, there are no wrong answers, and no one has to see what you write down. This activity is designed for you and you only, with the goal of helping you identify the emotions, events, and thought pattens that may be making you sick.

Why is it important to write down your answers? When you journal your feelings and thoughts, you pull the emotional pain, injury, and illness out of your body and put it down on paper. By doing so, you take these harmful emotions and thoughts out of you and bring them to light, where you can better understand them and begin to see them more objectively. You may have been allowing harmful emotions and thoughts to live rent-free in your body for years, but when you write them down, the act of journaling can help you realize that you don't have to let emotional trauma live inside you any longer. Journaling your answers and referring back to them over the next seven days and longer will also help remind you what you're working away from and what you want to eliminate, emotionally and spiritually, on your Day Seven during the Cleanse.

If Your Injury, Illness, or Condition Affects Your . . .

Brain: You may have an unwillingness or inability to look at your past.
    Ask yourself:

- Do I feel mostly at peace or am I upset with what has happened in my past?
- What memories or situations are the most difficult for me to remember or recall?
- Do I ever feel imprisoned by experiences or events in my past?

Heart: You may be suffering from unresolved grief.
    Ask yourself:

- What am I grieving that I've lost in my life?
- Do I share my grief with others or is it an isolated experience?
- In what ways is my grief preventing me from experiencing my life?

Throat: You may not be speaking your truth or feel silenced.
    Ask yourself:

- In what ways do I feel unheard or silenced in my life?
- What life experiences may have triggered a feeling of self-silence?
- Do I feel worthy of being heard?

Stomach: You may feel victimized or wounded or aren't able to acknowledge your power.

Ask yourself:

- How do I feel that I may be getting taken advantage of?
- Which areas of my life feel out of my control?
- Have I ever felt abandoned, isolated, or left behind?

Kidneys: You may be suffering from too much worry or anxiety.

Ask yourself:

- What am I scared of?
- How might fear be affecting my life?
- Do I feel more powerful than my worries or fear?

Liver: You may be suffering from or holding on to too much anger.

Ask yourself:

- What resentments am I hanging on to?
- How long have I felt angry?
- Do I feel angry more often than I feel peaceful?

Pancreas: You may be feeling too much responsibility or a lack of connectedness.

Ask yourself:

- Do I feel more or less connected to those around me on a daily basis?
- Do I feel like I'm always caring for other people?
- How often do I feel like other people don't understand me or can't relate to what I'm going through?

Blood: You may be resisting the natural flow of life.

Ask yourself:

- Do I feel like I'm thriving or simply surviving in life?
- In what areas of my life or in which ways do I restrict myself?
- Do I feel comfortable surrendering to the flow of life?

Skin: You may feel insecure about your image with others or have identity issues.
Ask yourself:

- What is my perception of how I am viewed by others?
- In what ways do I feel judged by people close to me or the outside world?
- What are my biggest fears about being truly seen?

Reproductive organs: You may have suffered sexual trauma or have identity issues with your gender.
Ask yourself:

- In what ways do I not feel at home in my sexual body?
- How do I view myself as a man or a woman?
- What issues have I experienced with sexual or romantic partners that make me feel uncomfortable or unworthy?

Bones: You may feel constrained by the structure of your life, including traditions, systems, or relationships you feel incapable of changing.
Ask yourself:

- In what ways do I feel confined by my own life?
- What traditions, relationships, or systems do I resent?
- How do I feel about changing certain traditions, relationships, or systems: hopeful or hopeless?

Spine: You may feel unable or have an inability to stand up for yourself.
Ask yourself:

- In what ways do I feel I may not be advocating for myself in my own life?
- How do I feel overlooked or unspoken for?
- What people, traditions, activities, or events make me feel powerless?

Shoulders: You may feel burdened or guarded.
   Ask yourself:

   - What might be causing me to feel overwhelmed or burdened?
   - Do I think that I'm not getting back what I give to others?
   - How are my feelings of being overwhelmed affecting my life?

Knees: You may feel unable or have an inability to move forward.
   Ask yourself:

   - What things in my past have I had trouble getting over?
   - In what ways have I not allowed myself to move forward or recover from past situations?
   - In what ways do I feel unbalanced or unable to stand on my own two feet?

Overcoming Emotional Trauma

After completing the preceding activity, you likely have a good idea of which negative emotions and thought patterns are keeping you from feeling better. Now it's time to work on addressing them so you can help your body heal and set yourself up for success on the Protocol.

Before we begin, it's important to realize and accept that no one can heal deep-seated emotional trauma or thought patterns overnight. These emotions and thoughts have been with you for a long time, and they'll take a while to dissolve. But making small, gradual changes to address them can lead to big shifts over time for your physical, mental, and emotional health.

I believe that the most effective way to address negative emotions and thought patterns is to replace them with positive ones. This may sound overly simple, but it works if you do the work. I use affirmations, which are positive statements that challenge negative emotions and thoughts. For example, if you discover that you feel powerless or are unable to stand up for yourself, you could use the affirmation, "I am in control of my life," or "I am courageous and deserve to be heard, seen, and respected." I recommend repeating affirmations out loud on a daily basis, as often as you can, to remind yourself of your worth, power, and/or potential to heal.

Why use affirmations? Research shows that self-affirmation activates the brain's reward centers that can limit pain and allow you to better navigate mental and emotional threats.[8] What's more, when you tell yourself the same thing over and over again, you write that information into both your body and your brain. In the brain, self-affirmation establishes new neural networks, which, over time, create new thought patterns.[9] These new thought patterns then trigger new biological processes, such as cell repair and growth. You can think of it like running, riding a bike, or swinging a golf club: When you repeat the same physical motions over and over again, it also creates new neural pathways in the brain that then establish new muscular memory and fine motor skills in your body. When you repeat the same positive words or thoughts over and over again, the same thing happens in the mind, with a correlative, positive effect on the body.

Like many psychologists, I believe any affirmations you create for yourself are more impactful, powerful, and empowering, because they're your words, personalized and tailored for your feelings. So, I suggest you sit down and brainstorm a set of affirmations of your very own that can help you counteract the negative emotions or thought patterns you identified in the preceding activity. The more specific you are, the more readily you will be able to pinpoint the negative thought patterns that need reversing.

Creating affirmations may come naturally to you, but if it doesn't, think about what you would tell your daughter, son, or best friend if you knew he or she was struggling with the same negative emotion or thought. Keep your affirmations short, positive—avoid using any negative words like *can't*, *don't*, or *won't*—and in the present tense. If you want, use a thesaurus to find more powerful words for what you want to say. Write your affirmations down in a journal or on sticky notes that you can attach to your kitchen cabinets, bathroom mirror, or bedside table to remind yourself to repeat them.

Self-affirmations alone, however, may not be enough to help you fully overcome negative emotions and thoughts. You may have to do some additional digging if you want to work through the harmful emotions that may be making you sick.

Exercise: How to Help Heal Emotional Trauma

The following activity complements the one you just completed to help you work through the harmful emotions and thoughts you now have identified. The instructions are the same: Carefully consider your answers to each of the three questions that pertain to any area of your body where you feel physically unwell. Write down whatever words, insights, or memories come to you without analyzing or judging them. If you find yourself stuck on a particular question, come back to it when you feel ready or have more mental clarity.

If Your Injury, Illness, or Condition Affects Your . . .

Brain: You may have an unwillingness or inability to look at your past.
Ask yourself:

- What old thoughts or beliefs could I revisit and use to help me heal?
- In what ways, large or small, can I allow myself to surrender one limiting thought at a time?
- In what ways, large or small, can I look at my past and release it on a daily basis?

Heart: You may be suffering from unresolved grief.
Ask yourself:

- What thoughts or beliefs could I use to help me release some of the sadness I'm holding on to?
- In what ways, large or small, can I open my heart on a daily basis?
- What thoughts make my heart feel heavy or burdened and how can I release them?

Throat: You may not be speaking your truth or feel silenced.
Ask yourself:

- What thoughts, beliefs, or words could I use to help me feel more heard?
- How can I find ways, large or small, to speak my truth every day?
- What words or phrases can I use on a daily basis to make me feel powerful?

Stomach: You may feel victimized or wounded or aren't able to acknowledge your power.

Ask yourself:

- What thoughts or activities make me feel powerful?
- Which thoughts or people in my life remind me that I'm not alone?
- In what ways, large or small, can I try to take back my power every day?

Kidneys: You may be suffering from too much worry or anxiety.

Ask yourself:

- What thoughts or beliefs trigger fear or anxiety in me?
- What thoughts or activities can I use to help me release worry?
- What new habits can I create to help me feel more safe and secure?

Liver: You may be suffering from or holding on to too much anger.

Ask yourself:

- What are the three primary sources of anger in life?
- In what ways, large or small, can I begin to release these sources of anger every day?
- What new thoughts or beliefs can I create to help me move from a place of anger to one of forgiveness?

Pancreas: You may be feeling too much responsibility or a lack of connectedness.

Ask yourself:

- In what ways have I isolated myself?
- In what ways, large or small, can I reconnect with those around me on a daily basis?
- What thoughts or beliefs might help me feel connected to my life and the world around me?

Blood: You may be resisting the natural flow of life.
Ask yourself:

- In what ways have I restricted my own joy or sense of fulfillment in life?
- What old thoughts or beliefs could I surrender that will help me trust the flow of life?
- What habits or thoughts can I create that could help me go with the flow more on a daily basis?

Skin: You may feel insecure about your image with others or have identity issues.
Ask yourself:

- In what ways can I let go of my fear of being judged?
- In what ways, large or small, can I heal my own insecurities?
- How can I find ways to love myself as I am?

Reproductive organs: You may have suffered sexual trauma or have identity issues with your gender.
Ask yourself:

- What thoughts or beliefs help me feel empowered in my sexuality?
- In what ways, large or small, can I release any shame I may have about my sexuality every day?
- What thoughts or beliefs am I ready to surrender about my sexuality?

Bones: You may feel constrained by the structure of your life, including traditions, systems, or relationships you feel incapable of changing.
Ask yourself:

- In what ways, large or small, can I create new structures and traditions in my life?
- What old thoughts or beliefs about the structure of my life can I release?
- The world around me is changing every day. In what ways can I change with it?

Spine: You may feel unable or have an inability to stand up for yourself.
Ask yourself:

- In what ways, large or small, do I already feel supported or can I feel supported?
- What new habits or thoughts can I adopt that might help me stand up for myself on a daily basis?
- In what ways can I release past memories of when I wasn't able to stand up for myself?

Shoulders: You may feel burdened or guarded.
Ask yourself:

- How can I relieve the small burdens in my life on a daily basis?
- Can I identify and let go of the burdens I may be carrying for others?
- In what ways, large or small, can I surrender or ask for help every day?

Knees: You may feel unable or have an inability to move forward.
Ask yourself:

- What thoughts or beliefs have kept me from moving forward?
- What goals or activities am I ready to move forward with?
- What new thoughts or activities, large or small, can I embrace on a daily basis?

If you've finished the exercises in this chapter, you've taken some amazing first steps to identify which emotions may be making you sick and to work toward replacing them with healthier feelings and thoughts. I suggest revisiting what you wrote down during the second exercise on a daily basis. Doing so will continue the work you've already started to replace negative emotions and thoughts with healthier, positive ones.

You don't have to spend hours every day thinking about how to make yourself emotionally healthier—just a few minutes can have a tremendous effect on healing harmful emotions and thoughts. Remember also to repeat your self-affirmations on a daily basis. Change won't happen overnight, but it *will* happen if you're consistent, patient, and positive.

In chapter 2, you learned that Day Seven is when your body is the most vulnerable. For this reason, I suggest you spend a few minutes before going to bed on Day Seven to say your affirmations and reread your answers to the questions completed in the second exercise. By focusing on creating healthier emotions and thought patterns before you go to bed, you'll set your body up to help eliminate negative feelings and thoughts during the final hours of the Cleanse instead of allowing them to take a deeper seat in the body.

CHAPTER 6

PREPARING FOR
AND PERSONALIZING
THE PROTOCOL

You're about to embark upon an incredible journey that will transform your body, mind, spirit, and soul. By following the day-by-day Protocol I'm about to detail in the next eight chapters, you'll learn how to adopt a lifestyle that will overhaul your health, energy, mental clarity, and emotional well-being. The way to true health and healing doesn't happen by forcing your body to do anything crazy, restrictive, trendy, or contrived but by doing just the opposite: The path to amazing health happens when you finally align your body with its age-old, universe-born, biological rhythms.

The Protocol has the potential to change not only your body but also your holistic sense of being. From the tips of your toes to the top of your head and inside out, nothing in your body is a static state: Whatever illness or ailment you have, you can change it, given the right circumstances. The most important part of any journey is always the decision to take the first step. This is the inflection point where intention meets action, where you form a synergy between your body, mind, and spirit, and where you create lasting, cathartic change. For this reason, I want to take a moment of pause and reflection so that you can become fully aligned with your intentions before you start.

I want to make sure you're entirely ready for the exceptional trip, with your bags packed with all the right stuff—not a snowsuit for the tropics or a swimsuit for the Alps. In practical terms, this means committing to certain goals, getting your head in the game, having realistic expectations, and learning to listen to what your body has been trying to tell you for years, since the day you were born. Here's what you need to know before you begin the Protocol:

Your individual issues are unique, but our priorities on the Protocol are universal—which is a good thing. Everyone reading this book will have slightly different illnesses or physical ailments they want to address, along with unique emotional traumas to overcome. But even though we all have our own unique physical issues and emotional traumas, we all have the same priorities on the Protocol: to sync with our universal and universe-given seven-day cycle to lower inflammation, eliminate toxins, traumas, and viral debris, and find newfound strength and empowerment in our natural biorhythms. We do this by eating the right foods at the right times, taking the right supplements on the right days, prioritizing how to move our bodies when it will most help our health, choosing when to let stress into our lives, and when to lean into allowing our bodies to relax and do what they need to do.

That we all have the same general priorities on the Protocol is a wonderful thing. It connects us all with each other and every other living person on the planet. The timing of our individual cycles may be slightly different depending on the day of the week on which we were born, but we all share the same opportunity and ancient power to take control of our health and healing.

Commit to the Protocol for *at least* **one week.** The Protocol only works if you adopt it for seven consecutive days. After all, the whole point of the Protocol is to align with your body's seven-day biological rhythms. Following the Protocol for anything less than seven consecutive days won't allow you to sync with your body's seven-day schedule. Think about it the same way you do antibiotics. You know that if you take a one-week round of antibiotics for anything less than seven consecutive days, the medication won't be able to do its job—you have to complete the full seven-day cycle in order for the drugs to kill all the harmful bacteria and fully heal you. The same is true of the Protocol.

What this means is that when you decide to start the Protocol, you should be ready to commit to it for *at least* one full week. For this reason, I suggest reading chapters 7 through 13 before you begin so that you know what to expect for each day of the week of the Protocol.

Think long term. You can definitely improve your health and energy by adopting the Protocol for one week only. But where the real transformations begin is after one month's time, which is how long I recommend you stick with the Protocol. Remember, I'm not asking you to undertake a restrictive diet, work out every day, or meditate for two hours daily—I just want you to align your life with your natural circaseptan rhythms.

It's just like syncing with your circadian rhythms, the body's twenty-four-hour internal clock. Let's say, for example, that you've been working the overnight shift for years, but your boss suddenly decides to change your schedule so that you work during the day. Great: Now you can finally wake up at a normal hour and go to bed before midnight, which studies show drastically reduces the risk of poor health associated with being out of sync with your circadian clock.[1]

But in this hypothetical scenario, if you adopted the day shift for twenty-four hours only, do you think you'd feel any better after one day? Of course not. If anything, you might feel less energetic because you just changed a pattern your body was accustomed to, even if that pattern was unhealthy. For real benefits, you'd need to stay in sync with your circadian rhythms for at least a few days straight before your energy, metabolism, mood, sleep, and other health parameters start to tick up in noticeable ways. The longer you're able to follow your circadian cycle, the healthier you'll be, too, since aligning with the body's twenty-four-hour clock is how we're all meant to live, getting up with the sun and going to bed shortly after it's dark.

The same is true of aligning with your seven-day cycle, except the stakes are much higher: After all, we're not talking about a 24-hour period but a 168-hour one. Syncing for one week will be helpful, but the longer you can sustain your seven-day cycle, the healthier you'll be—and the more noticeable results you'll see and feel. It's really that simple.

Slow and steady wins the race when it comes to health and healing. Getting on the Protocol isn't like swallowing a prescription drug: You won't feel incredibly different in an hour's time or even after one full day. Just like every other effective, sustainable, and truly healthy habit you can undertake, the Protocol works in gradual and cumulative ways.

But if you commit to the Protocol and follow it for at least one month, you will feel better—physically, mentally, emotionally, and spiritually. I see it all the time: A new patient or celebrity client adopts the Protocol, and one to two months later, my phone rings and it's that patient telling me how much better he or she feels and that X ailment or Y symptom finally went away. So take my advice: Give it at least one month, or four seven-day cycles. We'll talk more about how to maintain the Protocol in chapter 14, but in the interim, be patient and trust your body's process.

Make your goal to be good, not perfect. On the Protocol, I'm going to recommend that you prioritize some foods and do certain activities and types of exercise on specific days of the week while avoiding those things on others. I'm also going to suggest that you schedule certain medical procedures, treatments, and tests based on which day of the week it is.

But here's the deal: I know that regardless of how hard you try or how much you want to follow the Protocol to a T, you may not be able to move around an important work meeting, reschedule a cross-country flight, change the date of a child's birthday party, or delay surgery to better line up with your seven-day cycle. Similarly, a special occasion may come up when you want to celebrate with a cocktail or piece of cake on a day that isn't your six or seven.

That's all totally fine—life happens. But the most important thing you can do is try your best to live in sync with your seven-day schedule. You won't be able to do so every day of every week of every month of every year for the rest of your life, so aim for sustainability, not perfection—because the longer you can sustain the Protocol by making it work for you, the healthier and happier you'll be.

Stock up on supplements. In chapter 4, I detailed the list of supplements to take on the Protocol. It includes five specific, science-backed supplements to take Days One through Five to help your body heal and rebuild, along with three supplements for Days Six and Seven to help stimulate your liver to detoxify. You can also consider taking additional supplements Days One through Five if you're dealing with a thyroid issue, perimenopausal or menopausal symptoms, anxiety or depression, or a persistent viral infection like Lyme disease or Epstein-Barr virus. While the Protocol will work without supplements, taking them at the right times will effectively supercharge your body's best physiological processes. Think of it like different cars: Your body without the Protocol is like an old Model T, your body on the Protocol is like a contemporary sports car, and your body on the Protocol with supplements is like a Formula 1 race car—it will operate that much more efficiently. So before you begin the Protocol, go online or to your local health-food store and stock up on the supplements you need. This way, you'll be starting the program on Day One with all the bells and whistles that will maximize your results in less time.

Get your head in the game. You wouldn't show up to a big meeting with your boss or a relationship-defining talk with your partner without doing a little mental prep first. Similarly, you need to mentally prepare before you begin the Protocol. Make a mental commitment now to reset your body, initiate healing, and reverse whatever physical and emotional damage you may have been holding on to for years. Similar to how we tell our brains to move a body part before we can move—there's a millisecond of thinking that goes into every motion you make—we have to tell our brains to heal first in order to heal. Telling yourself that you're going to do something also establishes new neurons and pathways in your brain, which, over time, will become physiological actions in the body. For this reason, I recommend journaling what you want to accomplish or writing yourself a letter of intent. The more serious you take it, the more significant results you'll see and feel.

Have a conversation with your body. The Protocol is an amazing opportunity to get to know your body better and finally learn how to work in unison with your physical, emotional, and spiritual self rather than working against it—which is what most of us have done for years and years. This isn't your fault, of course—you didn't know about your body's seven-day schedule—but now that you've picked up this book, you have an opportunity to start listening to your body and what your organs, muscles, and cells have been trying to tell you since the day you were born. Now is the time to listen to your body's beautiful song and have a real conversation with yourself about who you are, where you've been, and where you want to go. Anything is possible on the Protocol. Now is the time for you and your body to accomplish what you've always wanted to do—together, in sync, and in rhythm with the universe that's both inside and all around you.

Personalizing the Protocol

Many patients see me because they've been battling a condition, illness, or disease for months or years with little to no improvement. They've been to many doctors and tried different drugs and treatments, but nothing gets better. These are the patients who are most excited to try the Protocol and do something—anything—to turn around how they feel or look. These are also my patients who have the most success alleviating or curing their condition, many times without the use of toxic pharmaceuticals or invasive surgeries.

Whether you want to lose weight, address hormonal issues, overcome a digestive ailment, reverse chronic pain, or combat cancer or an autoimmune disease, getting on the Protocol can help you treat or cure the problem. I've seen it happen over and over again with patients who had severe cases of the conditions listed in this chapter.

Adopting the Protocol and maintaining it for one month is step one. If you want to do everything possible to get results, consider customizing your seven-day cycle so that it better addresses your specific condition or concern. If you came to me as a patient, this is what I would do for you, tailoring the plan to your body, medical history, and individual health needs and goals. But in lieu of being able to see, listen, palpitate, and treat you in person, I want to give you the tools to personalize the Protocol as though we were working together in a one-on-one setting.

Before we get into the different conditions and how to customize the Protocol to best address them, I would encourage you to make an appointment with your primary-care doctor and ask for the following three tests. While none of these tests is mandatory, for some conditions, as you'll find noted over the next several pages, having testing done can help you and your doctor unlock what's really going on with your health and better treat your condition.

1. **A viral panel for Epstein-Barr virus (EBV) and cytomegalovirus (CMV):** These two viruses are extremely common in the general population. About 90 percent of all people become infected with EBV at some point during their lives[2] while 50 to 80 percent will develop CMV. When these infections are active, they increase inflammation, weaken the immune system, and can lead to the development of cancer and other degenerative diseases.[3] Knowing whether you have an active viral infection is paramount and can help you and your doctor better understand and treat your ailment. Just one note of advice: If you do test positive for EBV or CMV, consider seeing a naturopathic, integrative, or functional-medicine doctor who has the training or experience to treat the virus compared to conventional medicine practitioners.

2. **C-reactive protein (CRP) test:** This protein increases in the blood in the presence of inflammation, making it an easy way to assess your body's inflammatory load. If you have high CRP levels—generally considered to be more than 2.0 mg/L— I recommend committing to more than one month on the Protocol while maintaining a strict anti-inflammatory diet, taking all the supplements as recommended, and incorporating regular exercise, also shown to help lower CRP.[4] High CRP levels may also indicate the presence of a chronic disease or underlying inflammatory condition like cancer, lupus, inflammatory bowel disease, or rheumatoid arthritis, so it's a valuable test to get.

3. **Complete blood count (CBC) test:** This is Test 101 of basic blood work. CBC measures red and white blood cells, hemoglobin, hematocrit, platelet count, and other markers and is an easy, inexpensive, and low-effort way to get a quick snapshot of your general health. The test can also help

doctors diagnose a number of conditions, including anemia (low circulating iron), an infection, or a blood disorder.

Whether you choose to undergo testing or not, you can still personalize the Protocol to better treat your condition. Here, I've listed the twelve most common concerns or conditions I see in patients and what you can do to help address or cure them.

If You Want to Lose Weight . . .

Losing weight is as much about attitude as it is about what you put in your mouth on a day-to-day basis. How you view the food you eat, the ways in which you measure fat loss, and why you're trying to lose weight in the first place can dictate how successful you are independent of your diet.

Here's the first perception shift I recommend to anyone looking to lose weight: Throw away your scale. Body weight can fluctuate by five to ten pounds depending on your bathroom habits, exercise regimen, sodium intake, menstrual cycle, and how many carbs or cocktails you had the night before, in addition to other factors. If your weight doesn't change, or even if it ticks upward, you may be tempted to give up right when miracles are beginning to take place inside you. Instead of aiming to hit a specific number on the scale, make it your goal to feel better. If that's too vague or abstract, you can concentrate on whether your clothes fit better, you feel less bloated, and/or you feel lighter on your feet. If you need an objective marker of progress, track your fat loss using a measuring tape or body-fat calipers.

Second perception shift: Your primary goal should be to get healthy, not to lose weight per se. If you're unhealthy or out of sync with your natural seven-day rhythms, your body can't function optimally, making it very difficult to lose weight, no matter what you eat or how much you exercise.

Third perception shift: The Protocol is not a diet—it's an organic biorhythm and a natural lifestyle choice that uses foods, supplements, and daily habits to align how you nourish yourself with your body's seven-day cycle. When you sync your diet with your circaseptan rhythms, you improve your digestion, metabolism, inflammatory load, blood sugar levels, and body's ability to regulate its hormone production, all of which will help you to lose weight. While you'll want to minimize certain proinflammatory foods on the Protocol, especially added sugar and refined carbs, you don't have to cut them out completely, always and forever. Go ahead and eat what you crave no more than 20 percent of the time while making sure you're eating because you're hungry, not because you're bored, upset, or out of habit. I ask my weight-loss patients to make a list of five "treat foods" they can choose from to eat one at a time once a week, preferably on Day Five. For faster results, swap a traditional treat food for one with fewer inflammatory ingredients. For example, if your treat food is ice cream, look for a nondairy brand sweetened with stevia or monk fruit (all-natural sugar substitutes that don't contain any calories or sugar).

Why not cut out inflammatory foods completely? Studies show that exclusive or restrictive diets don't work in part because they cause people to feel deprived, which increases cravings and the likelihood to overeat or binge eat.[5] What's more, exclusive diets that eliminate foods or food groups are difficult to follow and can cause people to throw in the towel prematurely if they make even one misstep, which can also trigger feelings of failure, guilt, or shame.

If You Have Problems with Your Skin, Hair, or Nails . . .

Many patients who see me because they have dry skin, brittle hair, weak nails, or hair loss don't actually have problems with their skin, hair, or nails—instead they have hypothyroidism, a condition that occurs when the thyroid glands don't produce enough hormones. If you have a problem with your skin, hair, or nails, ask your doctor for a comprehensive thyroid panel that tests for free T3 and free T4. If any of your thyroid hormone markers are too low, talk to your doctor about treatment options and consider taking the supplements specified for those with thyroid issues Days One through Five.

Whether or not you have a thyroid problem, you can also supplement with biotin Days One through Five. Studies show this B vitamin, also found in some foods like eggs, beans, and nuts, increases keratin, a healthy protein found in skin, hair, and nails, and also regulates blood sugar to slow the body's inflammatory response to food.[6] In addition, I tell my patients to use only chemical-free skin- and hair-care products whenever possible, since toxins found in most conventional creams, lotions, shampoos, and conditioners can dry skin, hair, and nails and interfere with your body's natural growth cycle. Also look for skin-care products made with royal jelly or hair products made with tea tree or cannabidiol (CBD) oil, all of which have an anti-inflammatory effect.

If You Want to Sleep Better . . .

Sleep quality and quantity are multifactorial, influenced by many variables including diet, exercise, stress levels, prescription drug use, and alcohol consumption. If you have a sleep disorder or trouble falling asleep or staying there, I recommend doubling down on eating anti-inflammatory foods; exercising or moving your body at least five days a week; limiting your caffeine and alcohol consumption; learning to manage stress through meditation, yoga, and/or other modalities; and avoiding prescription sleeping pills. What's more, you should limit your exposure to the hormone-disrupting blue light emitted by computers and smartphones after 7 p.m.—if you continue to use these devices, all the sleep tips and tricks in the world won't help. At the same time, try to go to bed and wake up in the same two-hour window every night and morning.

I also recommend three supplements to patients with sleep problems. The first, melatonin, is a hormone produced by the body that helps induce sleep. For best results, take this supplement thirty minutes before you're ready for bed and then head for a dark room, which will help your body better synthesize the supplement. A second option is GABA, an amino acid and neurotransmitter that helps relax our neurological system. Known as "nature's Valium,"[7] GABA can be taken on an empty stomach, preferably one to two hours before dinner. The third supplement is CBD oil, which you should take immediately before bed. CBD, which contains no THC (the psychoactive chemical found in cannabis), has been shown to reduce anxiety, calm the nervous system, and promote feelings of general well-being.[8]

In addition to supplements, experiment with sleeping with white noise—try a box fan or download a special app for your smartphone—or weighted blankets. Both can help reduce anxiety and promote feelings of calm.

If You're Struggling with Low Energy or Fatigue . . .

If you're constantly tired or feel like you never have enough energy to do what you want, assess your sleep patterns and hygiene to make sure you're sleeping long enough and well enough. If you're not, see the preceding section on how to sleep better.

Chronic fatigue is a condition that mandates getting all three tests detailed on page 96 to make sure you don't have an underlying infection or illness that's sabotaging your body's ability to function. While you're at your doctor's, ask to have your iron levels and iron stores, or ferritin levels, tested—being low in either can cause anemia and exhaustion. Finally, opt for a B_{12} test: Many Americans are deficient in this nutrient, found only in animal foods, and suffer fatigue and mental health issues as a result.

I also tell my patients with low energy to exercise or move first thing in the morning. You don't have to run a 5K or even break a sweat, but moving for even fifteen minutes to raise your heart rate will also kick-start your metabolism, helping turn your brain on—and keep it on for the rest of the day. Before you eat breakfast, drink a cup of coffee or tea with a tablespoon or two of coconut oil or medium-chain triglyceride (MCT) oil; these healthy plant fats will stimulate your brain, which is 60 percent fat, helping to wake it up and get working. As you go throughout your day, be sure to drink enough water and eat high-fiber foods; being dehydrated or constipated can cause fatigue. Finally, limit the amount of time you wear sunglasses, especially in the morning, since the body uses photoreceptors in the eyes to help signal hormone production that dictate your energy and sleep-wake cycles.[9]

If You're Dealing with Chronic Pain . . .

I have great empathy for my patients with chronic pain who wake up hurting every day. For many, the pain becomes part of their identity and they resign themselves to living with it for the rest of their lives. While I understand how it's easy to feel a sense of hopelessness, I would encourage you to separate your pain from your body and see your suffering as a psychological problem rather than a physical one. Use the prompts on pages 80–83 in chapter 5 to name your pain outside of your body. For example, if you have pain in your shoulders, don't perceive it as a problem with your shoulders but as the emotional issue of feeling burdened. Or if you have knee pain, think of it as an inability to move forward. Use the mantras in that same chapter to help address these emotional blocks, based on which part of your body hurts.

Chronic pain is another condition that merits testing. Be sure to ask your doctor for a CRP test, which will show whether you have high levels of C-reactive protein, an inflammatory marker. In general, a CRP score above 2.5 mg/L indicates the presence of an illness, infection, or other inflammatory issue that could be causing chronic pain. I also recommend stretching or light movement first thing in the morning, even if you feel stiff. Raising your core temperature and increasing blood and nutrient flow will ease any stiffness and help lubricate and nourish your muscles and joints. You can also try taking an Epsom salt bath at least twice a week to help lower inflammation and calm your musculoskeletal system. Finally, remember to drink plenty of plain water to increase blood flow to painful areas, and minimize proinflammatory foods like added sugar, dairy, and refined carbs.

If You're Dealing with Hormonal Issues like Menopause, Low Testosterone, or Hypothyroidism . . .

In chapter 4, I detailed additional supplements you can take for thyroid issues and menopause or perimenopause symptoms. If you're dealing with any hormonal issue or imbalance, taking these supplements Days One through Five can make the difference between suffering through symptoms and feeling healthy and hormonally stable.

There are also other steps you can take to personalize the Protocol for hormonal issues. First, it's critical to reduce or eliminate the amount of animal meat you eat. Animal protein and fat contain naturally occurring hormones from the animal that can disrupt your body's hormonal balance when consumed in excess.[10] Synthetic hormones are also often added to conventionally raised animals to help increase their growth or dairy production. These hormones not only are toxic but also impact your body's ability to produce and regulate its own hormones.

Instead of animal meat, focus on consuming more plant protein and fat from nuts, beans, quinoa, avocado, and coconut oil. Your body needs nourishing plant fats to synthesize and regulate sex and thyroid hormones. If you're dealing with low testosterone, be mindful of soy, which can have an estrogenic effect on the body.

Unfortunately, animal meat isn't the only source of synthetic hormones. Most conventional personal-care products like antiperspirants, perfumes, lotions, shampoos, and creams contain chemicals that influence hormone production and regulation in the body. If you're dealing with any type of hormone issue, I'd recommend avoiding aluminum-based antiperspirant altogether and switching to all-natural, chemical-free skin- and hair-care products. Similarly, you'll also want to avoid chemical-based household cleaners—use all-natural products or a combination of water and vinegar instead—in addition to conventional gardening products, scented candles, and room sprays, all of which contain a high number of toxic chemicals.

If You're Struggling from Depression,
Anxiety, or Another Mental Health Issue . . .

If you're suffering from a mental health condition, seek professional help from a licensed therapist, psychologist, or psychiatrist. Mental health issues are common and affect people of all ages, incomes, education levels, personalities, and political parties, and there's nothing wrong with asking for help. While the Protocol can help stabilize mental and emotional health, I always recommend complementing it with professional treatment.

That said, there are many things you can do to shore up your mental health on the Protocol. First, I suggest getting your iron, ferritin, and B_{12} levels checked—being too low in any of these can cause mood problems. I also tell patients with depression or anxiety to exercise at least five days a week: Studies show physical activity is just as effective as prescription drugs in treating depression[11] and works the same way as antianxiety drugs like Xanax to calm the brain and ease tension, worry, and fear.[12] In addition, consuming foods like nuts, salmon, tofu, and eggs that are high in tryptophan—an essential amino acid that the body needs to manufacture the feel-good neurotransmitter serotonin—can help promote feelings of calm and stabilize mood.[13] You'll also want to limit your alcohol and caffeine intake, the latter of which can interfere with sleep—also critical for mood—and block the absorption of nutrients like magnesium, B_{12}, and vitamin D that play a key role in neurotransmitter production.[14]

Taking magnesium, B_{12}, and viatmin D in supplemental form can also help end unpleasant feelings while boosting mood. On pages 71–72 in chapter 4, I explained why taking B_{12} Days One through Five is essential for anyone with depression or anxiety. If you're serious about treating mental health issues, I'd also add magnesium to Days One to Five: Supplementing with the mineral has been shown to help treat major depression in just one week.[15] Taking vitamin D can also mitigate depression, anxiety, and seasonal affective disorder.[16]

Finally, I tell patients with mental health concerns to create a plan they can put into place whenever they feel depressed, anxious, lonely, or sad. My favorite recommendation is to move your body in any way: Take a five-minute walk around your neighborhood, do several minutes of jumping jacks and push-ups, or run through a quick yoga routine. If you suffer from anxiety, you can also try the five-four-three-two-one grounding technique: Identify five things you can see, touch four things, listen to three things (even if it's just your own voice or breath), smell two things, and taste one thing (even if it's only the inside of your mouth).[17] This exercise increases feelings of mindfulness and can make you feel safer and more grounded in your situation or surroundings.

If You Have Digestive Problems . . .

Inadequate muscle tone in the gastrointestinal tract—which is one giant muscle—can cause digestive problems, including bloating, heartburn, nausea, stomach pain, and constipation. One of the best ways to remedy the problem is to increase your intake of magnesium, in which half of all Americans are deficient. The mineral helps muscles to relax and contract so that your stomach can digest food more quickly and easily.

I also tell patients with stomach troubles to take probiotics. Research shows that supplementing with these healthy bacteria, which balance the body's microbiome, or the critical community of microorganisms that live inside the gut, helps to ease a range of digestive concerns.[18] If you've taken probiotics in the past with no effect, try again using a different product or strains (and preferably a supplement that needs to be refrigerated, since probiotics are living bacteria[19]): Studies show that probiotics work differently in different people, depending on your individual microbiome makeup.[20]

Taking supplemental aloe vera juice can also soothe your stomach and ease the acidic effect of many foods, doing for your GI tract what the calming plant does for skin after a bad burn. For best results, take aloe vera juice Days One through Five on an empty stomach in the amount recommended.

Finally, start your day with a big glass of warm water with lemon: The drink helps flush the GI tract, clearing undigested food particles and leftover debris that can irritate your gut and cause problems.[21]

If You Have Cancer . . .

Many patients come to see me because they've been diagnosed with cancer and find traditional treatment too toxic or not effective. The first thing I do with these patients is order a viral panel to determine whether they have an active EBV or CMV infection, both of which have been linked to cancer by the American Cancer Society.[22] If a patient tests positive, we focus their seven-day detoxification cycle on trying to eliminate the virus, making sure they supplement with lysine and cat's claw Days One through Five (see page 72 for why).

I also test cancer patients for genetic variants of the MTHFR gene, which helps the body process and use vitamin B_{12} and folate. MTHFR variants are extremely common, affecting more than half of all Americans.[23] While some variants are harmless, others can increase cancer risk, especially of the breast and ovaries.[24] If you're diagnosed with a variant, treating it is easy: You simply take methyl B_{12} and methyl folate—these supplements are more active, bioavailable forms of the vitamins—which help the body absorb the nutrients, obviating problems.

In addition, I recommend cancer patients supplement with lemon balm, already part of the Protocol Days One through Five, as research shows the herb helps kill cancer cells.[25] I also advocate using a form of medical marijuana, which will not only reduce symptoms associated with cancer and cancer treatment,[26] but may also limit tumor growth, according to studies.[27]

When it comes to diet, I tell patients to start the day by drinking some warm water with lemon to help flush viral debris that can develop in the GI tract overnight. Chase your lemon water with a green smoothie made from any green produce you like, such as spinach, kale, cilantro, cucumber, and green apple. Green fruits and veggies contain high amounts of chlorophyll, which studies show helps to reduce the spread of cancer.[28]

Finally, consider acupuncture Days Two through Five. The treatment, used in traditional Chinese medicine to treat liver stagnation, which is where cancer originates, can help ease symptoms and fight the disease.[29] Also, talk with your doctor about whether cryotherapy (extreme cold) or an infrared sauna might be right for you—both have been shown to boost immune function and suppress cancer growth.[30, 31] Acupuncture, cryotherapy, and infrared saunas are all complementary therapies to chemotherapy, radiation, and other conventional treatments for cancer. Still, be sure to speak with your acupuncturist, oncologist, or naturopath about the best way to incorporate these therapies into your treatment schedule.

If You Have Heart Problems . . .

If you have high cholesterol, blood pressure, or any other heart concern or condition, I recommend getting a specialized vertical auto profile (VAP), which can help identify the type, size, and density of the cholesterol particles in your blood. While some think the VAP test doesn't add much value, I believe the more you know about your body, the better you can tailor your treatment to your individual factors. Talk with your primary-care doctor, cardiologist, or naturopath about whether a VAP test is right for you. If you do get the test, work closely with a cardiologist or naturopath to interpret how the results might change your treatment. For example, a VAP test might show that you have a higher risk of heart disease than a regular cholesterol screening indicates or that your specific size or density of cholesterol warrants a different type of prescription drug or other intervention. Also, be sure to get a CRP test to identify whether base inflammation is causing or contributing to your condition.

In addition to testing, I also tell patients with heart conditions to supplement with magnesium, which studies show lowers blood pressure and mental stress while helping the heart muscle better contract and relax.[32] Take the mineral Days One through Five, along with CBD, which research has found can help reduce inflammation.[33] Finally, talk with your doctor about how you can safely add more exercise to your daily or weekly routine: Moving your body for just ten minutes a day can lower your risk of dying from heart disease by 33 percent, according to studies.[34]

If You Have Diabetes or Prediabetes . . .

For patients with type 2 diabetes or prediabetes, I suggest getting a candida screen to determine whether a yeast overgrowth is causing or worsening their condition. Research shows that candida in the GI tract can trigger insulin resistance.[35] At the same time, people with diabetes are more likely to develop yeast overgrowths or infections,[36] so it's important to treat a yeast problem if you have one.

When it comes to supplements, consider taking two tablespoons of apple cider vinegar before bed, which studies show lowers blood sugar in people with type 2 diabetes.[37] You can also try taking the same dose after meals, which research shows can help regulate blood sugar.[38] There's strong research showing that zinc supplements can also lower blood sugar and help diabetics better manage the condition.[39] Another mineral to supplement with is chromium, which many people don't consume enough of. For those with diabetes, the mineral has been shown to lower blood sugar and reduce insulin resistance.[40]

Exercise is also key to prevent and treat insulin resistance,[41] as is regular acupuncture Days Two through Five, which can help lower blood sugar and improve insulin sensitivity.[42]

Autoimmune diseases, including rheumatoid arthritis, lupus, psoriasis, Hashimoto's disease, and irritable bowel disease, occur when the body's immune system starts to attack healthy tissue. Both EBV and CMV infections can lead to autoimmune disorders, so getting a viral panel that can test for an active infection is critical. If you test positive, take lysine and cat's claw Days One through Five, as indicated on page 72.

Those with autoimmune diseases should also be tested for the MTHFR gene variant, which is associated with autoimmune conditions.[43] If you have a variant, supplement with methyl B_{12} and methyl folate. Even without a variant, consider taking a B complex to help improve energy, which is often low in those with autoimmune diseases. Cannabis or CBD supplements can also help lower inflammation and reduce symptoms associated with the conditions.[44]

One of the most effective ways to combat autoimmune diseases is with exercise. While many with autoimmune disorders aren't physically active or don't believe they can be due to neurological or musculoskeletal symptoms, engaging in some sort of muscle reflex therapy will boost immune function and reduce the likelihood of autoimmune attacks, according to research.[45]

DAY ONE: NEW BEGINNING

CHAPTER 7

I have three kids. And like any mother who's experienced the pain and joy of childbirth, I know that the day an infant is born is one of the most difficult for both you and your baby. But the day after your child is born? That's a magical moment. It often feels as though you've entered the calm after a storm, like a whole new world has broken open for both you and your baby. The trauma is over, and while you're both exhausted from the effort, energy, and chaos of childbirth, there's a quiet and peaceful sense that this is the start of something new and amazing.

I experienced this with all three of my children. When my oldest son, Tucker, was born, for example, I had to have an emergency C-section. While Tucker didn't have to go through the trauma of being squeezed out the birth canal, getting ripped from my abdomen was no picnic, either. Suddenly, my tiny son was in the bright, cold, chaotic world of real life, where his body had to function on its own in seconds to survive. This is the most traumatic transition our bodies ever endure, and Tucker remained overly distressed and agitated for hours afterward. He cried constantly and couldn't get comfortable or lie with me in bed. He slept very erratically in his bassinet the first night, where hospital nurses checked on him every twenty minutes.

The next day, though, Tucker was an entirely different baby: calm, happier, and healthier. He no longer cried constantly or tried to wriggle out of any position we put him in, and he started sleeping with me. He also began to breastfeed, and when he wasn't sleeping or feeding, he remained alert, not clouded or inconsolable.

I keep coming back to the idea that Day One is the calm after the storm: the day the dust settles and you begin to reemerge after your body's most tempestuous time. It's also a new beginning: the day when your body resets and starts its seven-day cycle all over again. This makes Day One an opportunity for reinvention and metamorphosis, when you can decide to reshape your body, mind, and spirit into whatever you want them to be.

Biology: What Happens in Your Body Today

From a biological perspective, your body responds similarly on Day One to how Little Newborn You did the day after you were born. You've just lived through the Cleanse—the weekly reoccurrence of your birth—when your body culminated its seven-day cycle of inflammation and detoxification. Your levels of inflammatory markers, toxins, and viral debris were sky-high yesterday, and while your body has worked arduously to try to flush them, not everything leaves your blood and lymphatic system the moment the clock ticks past midnight on Day Seven.

From the blood results of hundreds of patients and clients, I've estimated that the liver can clear around 90 percent of measurable inflammation and toxins by Day One, meaning 10 percent are still floating around inside. What this means is that while the Cleanse of your Day Seven may be over, your body is still working (albeit much less frantically) to flush any remaining inflammation and waste.

While your body continues to detoxify on Day One, your hormones begin to reregulate, as levels of estrogen, testosterone, and cortisol, the body's stress hormone, drop after their weekly peak. Midway into Day One, all the neurotransmitters that your body produced in response to Day Seven's trauma—our fight-or-flight chemicals, including dopamine, norepinephrine, and epinephrine (adrenaline)—start to fall. Your neurological system also begins to relax, making you less sensitive to light and sound. At the same time, your executive function, including your ability to plan, focus, make decisions, and handle emotions, sharpens, as your brain is no longer clouded by inflammation and excess hormonal and neurotransmitter activity.

There is one neurotransmitter, however, that doesn't drop on Day One: serotonin. We actually begin to produce *more* of this feel-good chemical on Day One, as the gut, responsible for manufacturing 90 percent of all serotonin in the body,[1] becomes less inflamed. This boost in serotonin is one reason many feel calmer on Day One.

A less inflamed gut has other benefits in addition to mood. As the lining of your gut begins to heal, you can also start to feel less bloated. Your body will also be able to absorb more nutrients from food and supplements, too.

In addition to the brain and gut, every other organ in the body begins to return to baseline on Day One after being thoroughly taxed and depleted Days Six and Seven. This includes your liver and kidneys—the two organs primarily responsible for detoxifying the body. Your liver enzymes drop dramatically on

Day One—something I saw over and over again in patients' blood work—along with your white blood cell count, which increases Days Six and Seven in response to elevated inflammation. Your blood pressure and heart rate also normalize, as the fascia, or the connective tissue surrounding your muscles and organs, begins to relax. These physiological effects, in conjunction with increasing serotonin, can contribute to the sense of relief or even serenity many feel on Day One.

Physically, you should feel better on Day One than you did on Day Seven. But don't expect to wake up feeling like a million bucks—you're definitely still in recovery mode. You should think of yourself as a newborn baby and treat yourself like one, too. Your Day One is a day to create a new intention and foundation for your week.

Emotions: What Happens in Your Mind Today

It's normal to wake up feeling a little lost or even empty today. The Cleanse the day before can cause many people to feel depleted or even hollow inside. You may also feel some residual anger, irritability, or frustration leftover from the elevated hormones, neurotransmitters, and inflammatory markers surging through your body on Day Seven. At the same time, it's not unusual to feel expectant, hopeful, and even optimistic, as your body begins to embark upon a brand-new seven-day cycle.

No matter what you're feeling today, take the time to acknowledge your emotions and that your heart and spirit may need as much coddling Day One as your body does. Be gentle with yourself and be positive about your health, life, and overall outlook: What you think, feel, and believe today can work wonders to ingrain new patterns that will shape what happens in your body and mind for the rest of your seven-day cycle.

Daily Mantra: What to Tell Yourself to Stay Centered and Help Heal

Having a daily mantra can help ground you, make you more mindful of your body and its biorhythms, and increase your mind-body-spirit connection. Setting a purpose for each day can also help provide extra determination to focus on your daily mantra and actions. To drive home today's purpose, remember that you're taking a first step in your healing journey—it doesn't matter how big or small the step is. Repeat the mantra when you wake up and whenever you feel uncentered or uncertain throughout the day.

I have the power to heal within me.

Actions: Best Things to Do Today

1. **Make more time.** The name of the game on Day One is easy does it. If you can, allow yourself to sleep in a little later-you'll have the next several days to jump out of bed and carpe diem-and give yourself some extra time to get ready in the morning. The same is true of today's schedule: Day One is not the time to pack your agenda with meetings, appointments, and social obligations from sunup to sundown. Similarly, if you're working under a deadline or with certain expectations today, build in a little wiggle room to allow yourself to get everything done. While you may have more mental clarity and higher executive function today, you're still reeling-physically, mentally, and emotionally-from higher inflammation and the Cleanse.

2. **Take inventory, make lists, and set goals.** Day One is a new beginning and fresh start-it's your body's equivalent of a clean slate. That makes today ideal to take inventory of where you are in life, along with what you want to do and where you want to go. Journal your thoughts or make a list of what you have or what you want to accomplish. This is a great day to set goals and intentions or to create a vision board, which you can do by compiling images (photographs, magazine cutouts, drawings, your own artwork) on a poster-size board that you can mount in a visible place.

3. **Plan, but don't necessarily do.** Day One is ideal for organizing, scheduling, and planning but not necessarily for doing, as your body is still recovering from the Cleanse. I suggest you use the day to plan meetings, schedule appointments, meal prep, and organize the week ahead.

A WEEK TO CHANGE YOUR LIFE

4. **Minimize stressful situations.** Since your body is still recouping from Day Seven, today is not a good day to introduce anything stressful–remember, you're like a newborn baby who needs to be coddled and cared for. I always tell my celebrity clients not to read new movie reviews or gossip websites on Day One, since doing so, if the content is negative, could send their stress levels soaring again–the last thing you want on Day One. Similarly, today is not the time to have a tête-à-tête with your spouse or boss or send any emails that may elicit a stressful response.

HEALTH: MEDICAL TESTS, TREATMENTS, AND THERAPIES TO PRIORITIZE TODAY

1. **Start a new medication.** Day One is the body's beginning, so now is the time when you'll be most receptive to integrating any new drugs or medication. Since your body is a proverbial clean slate, it's highly receptive to accepting new inputs and making them part of your seven-day cycle.

2. **Adopt a new diet or other healthy habit.** Day One is also ideal to begin a new diet or any other healthy habit that requires changing intentions or behaviors. You're physiologically and mentally more receptive to new things–and any patterns you establish today have the highest chance of being adopted and ingrained in your seven-day cycle.

3. **Do intravenous treatment.** Your body just got rid of a lot of inflammation, toxins, and viral debris, which means there's more room in your blood and lymphatic system for medication or other therapies administered intravenously.

4. **Schedule your tests.** I don't recommend that anyone have blood work or other diagnostic testing today unless absolutely necessary, as your body is still clearing remaining toxins, which

can obscure results. Instead, use the time to schedule these tests, along with any other medical appointments.

SELF-CARE: BEST WAYS TO NOURISH YOUR BODY, MIND, AND SPIRIT TODAY

1. **Meditate.** Every day of the Protocol is a good day to meditate. But practicing mindfulness today is especially effective since the brain is a blank slate and thereby most receptive to creating healthier new neural pathways–connections in the brain that studies show can be forged by regular meditation.[2] These connections, in turn, can become permanent new ways of thinking and coping, as your brain ingrains whatever you do or think today into your seven-day cycle. Taking the time to meditate today also gives you a chance to find a quiet moment to reflect on the trauma of Day Seven. Because today is also a good day for goal setting, meditation can help you visualize any goals you set for yourself.

2. **Stretch.** When we move our muscles, ligaments, and tendons, studies show it helps move lymphatic fluid, along with the waste products it contains, through the body.[3] While exercise is great for lymphatic drainage (more on this on page 115), stretching can be uniquely beneficial by helping to loosen tight muscles that may be preventing lymphatic flow. Try dynamic stretching, or using movement to elongate muscles, by doing leg swings, shoulder shrugs, neck rotations, arm circles, ankle pumps, and similar exercises.

3. **Try dry brushing.** This age-old Ayurvedic technique, which involves rubbing skin with a stiff-bristled brush, helps promote blood flow and lymphatic drainage, according to major medical institutions.[4] To try it yourself, invest in a large shower or bath brush with natural coarse bristles. Beginning at your ankles, brush your skin with gentle, fluid, circular strokes, working upward until you've scrubbed your entire body. Shower

afterward to remove any dead skin cells and toxins released from open pores.

Laura's Story: The Power of Day One

I want to tell you about my patient Laura. What happened to her on her Day One isn't typical per se, but her story exemplifies the power of the Protocol and Day One specifically as a new beginning for the body, mind, and spirit.

Five years ago, Laura was married, living in a fancy uptown apartment in New York City, and working as CEO of one of the top telecommunication companies in the world. She seemed to have it all, including a salary that distinguished her as one of the highest-paid female executives in the country. But what Laura didn't have, despite all the power, prestige, and money, was happiness.

Laura started seeing me for a fairly uncomplicated reason: She was struggling with some symptoms of menopause and wanted to get her hormones under control. But after a few weeks on the Protocol, she discovered that there was something greater that she wanted to get under control—her life. She began to confront old emotional trauma and uncover a new level of physical and mental clarity. This clarity grew and grew until, exactly four weeks into the Protocol, Laura woke up and quit her job, chopped off her hair, filed for divorce, and announced that she was moving to Bali. And she did this on the day of all days for new beginnings: her Day One. It's the time when the fog clears from the windshield and we can see the road before us—and Laura didn't like what she saw.

The truth was, Laura hadn't realized how unhappy she had become. First, there was her job. While the fifty-five-year-old had enjoyed an impressive career on paper, she had never felt fulfilled—telecommunications had never been her life's passion. Next, there was her marriage. She knew her husband had been having affairs for years, but she had been willing to overlook them because they were an influential couple in one of the country's most high-society cities. But as she went through the physical and emotional work of the Protocol, she realized that she was tired of living a lie, especially since the rewards of doing so only meant a routine of unsatisfying social parties and a loveless marriage.

As for her hair, for Laura this was another symbol of the costume disguising the authentic self she craved. It was long, lifeless, and styled just so in order to fit in with what people expected of a high-powered corporate woman working in a man's world. She didn't like it, and she never had.

After following the Protocol for four weeks, Laura woke up on Day One with a clearer mind and strong drive for renewal and rebirth. She hadn't necessarily planned to quit her job that day—she was still working out details of when and how—but as the fog cleared and she could suddenly see the road before her, she knew she couldn't wait any longer for her life to start.

The first thing Laura did was take the subway (not a cab) to her office in Midtown, where she told the director of the board that she was stepping down. She then got back on the subway, taking it downtown this time to a new salon she had heard her younger assistants gushing over. She didn't have an appointment and asked for the first stylist who was free—a young woman in her twenties with pink hair and flower tattoos up and down one arm. Laura told the stylist simply to cut her hair off, and the young woman, empowered by her client's confidence and trust, grinned and clipped Laura's hair into a pixie. Laura looked in the mirror and smiled.

Feeling freer, sexier, and suddenly happier, Laura hailed a cab back uptown to her attorney's office. She had thought about it for years, but now she was finally ready. She signed the papers and told her lawyer to serve her husband for divorce.

There was just one more thing to do: Laura wanted to tell those she cared about that she'd be moving in a month to Bali. She went home, picked up the phone, and starting dialing—I was one of several who got the call that day. And the more people she called, the more it set in: Laura wasn't just starting a new seven-day cycle—she was starting a new life.

One year later, when I spoke to Laura on the phone again, she was still living in Bali and still sporting her pixie cut. She also had a boyfriend and a small restaurant, which had been a dream of hers for years. Today, a full five years later, she's still living on the island and tells me she's happier than she's ever been.

Laura's story is extraordinary, I know. By no means do you need to, nor should you, use the Protocol to quit your job, end a relationship, or overhaul your entire life in a single day unless that's what you want to do. And while Day One isn't necessarily the best day to make decisions on the Protocol—that's Days Two through Four, when you have basement-low inflammation and more cognitive and emotional clarity—Laura's story is the perfect example of what can happen when we get in line with our bodies and finally shed old physical, mental, and emotional baggage that may have held us down for years.

EXERCISE: BEST WAYS TO MOVE YOUR BODY TODAY

1. **Focus on fluid movements.** Gentle exercise like yoga, Pilates, tai chi, walking, swimming, and golfing is one of the best ways to stimulate the body's lymphatic system to flush any remaining toxins and waste. Since your lymphatic system doesn't have a major organ like the heart to pump fluid and waste, moving your body will increase muscle movement, blood flow, and heart rate, all of which can help keep lymphatic fluid flowing and eliminate toxins, according to research.[5] If you like to swim, pool run, or do water aerobics, today is ideal for water exercise, since the combination of water pressure and physical activity is extremely effective for increasing lymphatic flow and drainage.

2. **Avoid intense workouts.** While intense workouts can be super healthy for your body and brain at times, they won't do you any favors on Day One. That's because intense and/ or jarring sports like running, heavy weight lifting, CrossFit, mixed martial arts, boxing, football, basketball, lacrosse, and mountain biking increase inflammation—and since your body just spent two days in a highly inflamed, overtaxed state, adding more inflammation today will only impair your ability to heal and start fresh. Save these sports for later in the week when your body can better handle the stress load and will be receptive to the aerobic and anaerobic benefits of high-intensity exercise.

3. **Keep it under an hour.** Exercising for long periods of time can also inflame your body and increase levels of the stress hormone cortisol. Cap your aerobic workouts on Day One to an hour to keep your body on its recovery path. Focus on stretching instead or adopting the aforementioned fluid movements.

Supplements: Best Nutrients to Take
to Support Your Body and Mind Today

In chapter 4, we talked about creating a ritual around taking your supplements in order to help you not only get into the habit but also increase their efficacy. Remember that if you believe that something will work and visualize it taking effect, it has a much greater chance of doing so. When you take your supplements today, I want you to visualize that you're planting five fresh seeds of health, growth, and wellness in the fertile soil of your body.

- Turmeric
- Wheatgrass
- Probiotics
- Royal jelly
- Lemon balm

Those with thyroid issues can take the following supplements in the morning, according to package instructions:

- Vitamin B_{12}
- Cat's claw
- Methylfolate

Those experiencing menopausal or perimenopausal symptoms can take the following supplements in the morning, according to package instructions:

- Red raspberry leaf extract
- Methylfolate

Those with depression or anxiety can take the following supplements in the morning, according to package instructions:

- Vitamin B_{12}

Those who have a viral infection (acute or chronic) can take the following supplements in the morning, according to package instructions:

- Lysine
- Cat's claw

The Best Thing to Drink Today

Prioritizing water on the Protocol is always important, but drinking more H_2O today will help flush remaining toxins from the Cleanse. While any water is better than soda, sports drinks, juice, or other sugary or artificially sweetened beverages, there's one type of water that will do double time for your body and overall health today: Studies show that drinking alkaline water, which has a higher pH than regular tap water, can help neutralize acid in the blood, helping to lower any residual oxidative stress from yesterday's Cleanse.[6] You can find alkaline water in most supermarkets—look for labels from major brands like Icelandic and Smartwater—or make it at home using special filter sticks or water pitchers with built-in alkaline filters.

Diet: Best Foods to Prioritize Today

The following eight foods promote lymphatic drainage, helping to encourage your body to get rid of any remaining toxins, waste, and viral debris from Day Seven:

- Spinach
- Ground flaxseed
- Chia seeds
- Brazil nuts
- Garlic
- Cranberries
- Walnuts
- Avocados

DAY TWO: BACK TO BASELINE

I f Day Seven is the storm, Day One is like the calm after the storm, when everyone is out on the streets, sweeping up the mess, chatting with their neighbors, and taking in all the sunshine and fresh air after being cooped inside for days. If we turn this analogy into biology, Day Two is when your body goes back to normal after the storm: Everything is bright and still, nothing is increasing or building, and any remaining inflammation or toxins from your body's big purge on Day Seven have finally been cleared. Your body basically just is. And for this reason, you're better able to appreciate all the sunlight and fresh air of life right now.

Day Two is one of the biggest windows of opportunity we have all week to overhaul our health and bodies' ability to heal. That's because inflammation is lowest today than it'll be at any other point in our seven-day cycle—and if we can drive that inflammation down even farther today, we can effectively reset our inflammatory baseline for the rest of the week. So instead of beginning your body's seven-day buildup of inflammation at a five on a hypothetical scale from zero to ten, you could start at a two. This means you'd limit just how inflamed your body can be on Day Seven, making the Cleanse less of a traumatic event for both you and your body. Less inflammation for the week also means you'll have more energy, look and feel better, and be able to more effectively fight off illness or any other ailments caused by inflammation.

There's another advantage to your body's rock-bottom inflammation levels today, too. When your brain and blood aren't clouded by hormones, toxins, and other inflammatory markers, you're able to focus and find mental clarity. You're also more emotionally stable and less likely to be agitated, irritable, or stressed today than any other day of the week. The way I look at it, the water flowing all around us is crystal clear on Day Two, and we can see everything in fresh, distinct colors, including our own reflections. Mentally and emotionally, we're functioning optimally, which makes today an ideal time for those challenging conversations or big meetings you may have put off the last few days. From a physiological perspective, since we have super-low inflammation levels, any forms of acute inflammation we incur from things like intense workouts will benefit our bodies rather than harm them.

In short, Day Two is all about enjoying your body in its simplest, healthiest form: clear, calm, open, and ready. Here's how to take advantage of everything today has to offer and help turn you at baseline into a healthier and happier person.

Biology: What Happens in Your Body Today

I see it all the time when I take blood from patients on Day Two: Nearly every inflammatory marker, including certain hormones, enzymes, and proteins, is the lowest today than I'll see in the same patient all week. Their levels of estrogen, testosterone, and the stress hormone cortisol are all flat, along with their liver enzymes and white blood cell count. Their bodies have finally cleared all the toxins and viral debris from their blood, liver, and lymphatic systems, and things like cytokines and C-reactive protein that are elevated when we're stressed or inflamed are nowhere to be found.

The body's histamine levels are also at an all-time low today. You probably know what histamines are if you've ever had an allergic reaction: These chemicals trigger the immune system to react to any possible allergen, causing you to sneeze, itch, or tear up in order to get the irritant out of your body or off your skin. But having high histamine levels can also cause inflammation. Because histamines are stored in the liver, which just underwent its big purge on Day Seven, your levels are low today.

Because histamine and inflammation levels are so low today, your immune system is not on high alert, as it is Days Six and Seven, when the body is building up inflammation and detoxifying. Instead, your T cells, which the immune system releases to attack toxins and other foreign substances in the body, don't have any internal trauma to respond to today, allowing them to function proactively and target latent chronic illness or disease.

Your blood is also more oxygenated today than it will be all week, due to lower levels of cortisol, inflammation, and viral debris. More blood oxygen means better blood flow, helping your heart, liver, and other internal organs receive more nutrition today. Your joints and muscles also benefit from more oxygenated and better-flowing blood, which is why you may feel less soreness, stiffness, and pain than you will all week.

Emotions: What Happens in Your Mind Today

I love working with people on Day Two because it's usually when they feel the greatest sense of mental focus and clarity—nothing is building up, purging, or otherwise distracting your body or brain. After a few weeks on the Protocol, many patients tell me that they discover this heightened clarity on Day Two helps them finally realize what's been standing in their way or holding them back from being truly happy or healthy. Day Two can be eye-opening, and I encourage you to be receptive to whatever you may see in your body, mind, and spirit today.

It's not unusual to feel some peace, contentment, and even gratitude today. Your body has returned to baseline and a place that feels really good, and this can sometimes stimulate a sense of closure and satisfaction.

This doesn't mean that things will always be bright and sunny on Day Two. After all, what's happening in your body doesn't always dictate what happens in the outside world. You have the same chance today as any other day of getting bad news, experiencing something traumatic, or being treated poorly. The only difference, though, is that if something negative or harmful does occur today, you'll be able to respond more effectively or calmly than any other day of the week.

Daily Mantra: What to Tell Yourself to Stay Centered and Help Heal

To drive home today's purpose, know that you have the clarity to separate what energy is your own and what belongs to other people or external demands. Repeat the following mantra when you wake up and whenever you feel uncentered or uncertain throughout the day:

I don't have to take on any drama or negative energy that isn't my own.

Actions: Best Things to Do Today

1. **Seize the day.** Your body and mind are functioning optimally today, with lower levels of inflammation and oxygen than at any other point in your seven-day cycle. I always tell my patients not to waste this amazing opportunity by spending the day in bed, watching Netflix, or having a spa day—that's

what Days One, Six, and Seven are for. Day Two is when you should try to jump out of bed and aim to accomplish whatever you set your mind or heart to doing.

2. **Challenge yourself.** Put all the mental clarity and emotional stability you have today to work by scheduling a test, delivering a high-pressure presentation, or performing in any other way, whether it's personal or professional.

3. **Travel.** If you have flexibility in your schedule, try to book any long flights, car rides, or other substantial travel for Day Two. Since inflammation is so low today, your body will bounce back quickly from the stress of travel, and you should experience less jet lag, muscle stiffness, and other detrimental effects.

4. **Have that stressful conversation.** With good mental clarity, emotional stability, and a sharper sense of self today, now is the ideal time to have those confrontational or potentially stressful conversations that you should otherwise try to minimize on Days One, Six, or Seven.

HEALTH: MEDICAL TESTS, TREATMENTS, AND THERAPIES TO PRIORITIZE TODAY

1. **Do blood work.** Today is the day when our blood is the clearest, unclouded by the inflammatory markers, toxins, and other waste products that the body naturally produces and expels. If you have to have your blood drawn, try to schedule the appointment for Day Two. Not only will your results be more accurate but if you happen to have something malignant in your body, your doctor should be able to identify it more readily in blood drawn on Day Two, when other markers won't obscure the results.

2. **Undergo diagnostic imaging.** With less inflammation and other junk in your body, today is the ideal time for any imaging tests like MRIs, CT scans, and mammograms. If you can schedule

these tests for Day Two, you'll get the clearest picture, helping your doctor better diagnose or discern any problem areas.

3. **Schedule that invasive procedure.** If you have to have surgery, a planned C-section, or any other type of invasive procedure, Day Two is one of the best days to do it. Less inflammation, more oxygenated blood, and an army of proactive immune cells can help increase the likelihood of a successful procedure while minimizing your recovery time.

Julie's Story: The Power of Day Two

At age forty-five, Julie was concerned that she had already run out of options. It had been three months since she had been first diagnosed with stage IV breast cancer, and the disease wasn't responding at all to the treatment she was receiving at Brigham and Women's Hospital in Boston—one of the best medical facilities in the country. Her oncology team now worried that her cancer was more aggressive than they had originally hoped, as the disease showed no signs of abating after several cycles of chemotherapy and radiation. Each week, her doctors increased her dose, and it was almost time, they told her, to start looking at more invasive therapies. This is when Julie called me.

When I met with Julie, she was desperate, fearful that she wouldn't live long enough to see her eleven-year-old son graduate from high school. Under different circumstances she might not have been so amenable to the Protocol, but she was now at the end of her rope and willing to try anything to keep from falling off. When I suggested to Julie that she have imaging and blood work done only on her Day Two, when her body's natural seven-day cycle of inflammation wouldn't cloud her results, she didn't hesitate. I also asked her to cut sugar and refined carbs, red meat, cow's dairy, nightshade vegetables, and corn from her diet, while taking all the supplements outlined in chapter 4.

Julie didn't tell her doctors why she wanted to start having weekly blood draws and monthly imaging on Wednesdays only—her Day Two. I also suggested she line up her chemotherapy to take place on Days Five and Six, when her body was preparing to detoxify, to help mitigate the harmful effects of the drug.

After just one Wednesday of blood work, Julie's doctors called her with the good news: Both her liver enzymes and white blood count were much lower, and her overall liver and kidney function had improved. Three weeks later, when she finally had an MRI on a Wednesday, her doctors had a much different prognosis than they had since she first started her treatment: Her cancer was finally responding. They could see her tumor more clearly, and it appeared to be beginning to shrink.

One month after Julie changed her testing to take place only on Wednesdays, her doctors had even better news: Her cancer was now responding so well that they wanted to begin to level off her chemo and eventually reduce her dosing of the toxic medication. When I asked Julie how her oncologists explained her sudden and significant turnaround, she told me that they said she must previously have had white-coat syndrome—a medical term for when a fear of doctors, hospitals, or medical procedures can increase your blood pressure, cortisol, and other biological markers related to anxiety. While Julie's cortisol and other hormone levels could have technically been higher due to white-coat syndrome, there was no way even the greatest degree of fear or anxiety could have caused her blood cell counts and liver and kidney function to indicate that her cancer wasn't improving. Instead, Julie and I both knew her turnaround had nothing to do with fear and everything to do with the Protocol.

Six months later, Julie ended chemotherapy treatment altogether, and we began working with her body's seven-day cycle to detox the medication and heavy metals from her body. That was five years ago, and Julie has been in remission ever since. Today, she credits syncing her testing and treatment with her body's natural rhythms as the game changer in her fight against cancer.

SELF-CARE: BEST WAYS TO NOURISH YOUR BODY, MIND, AND SPIRIT TODAY

1. **Practice breath work.** You can enhance and deepen your mental clarity today by practicing breath work, which will bring even more oxygen into your brain and bloodstream. When doing breath work, I like to use fellow naturopath Dr. Andrew Weil's four-seven-eight technique: Breathe in through your nose for a count of four, hold your breath for seven, then exhale through your mouth for a count of eight. Repeat several times, or until you feel calmer and more mentally energized.

2. **Try something new.** Your mind and heart are in a place today where they will react very positively to any new challenges or stimulation you provide. If there's something you've always wanted to try, learn, or say, today is the day to push yourself to do it.

3. **Read.** With increased focus, you'll absorb more of what you read today than any other day of the week. Prioritize time for a good book or try to tackle a more complicated or obtuse piece of reading that you've been putting off.

EXERCISE: BEST WAYS TO MOVE YOUR BODY TODAY

1. **Run.** Going for a jog can trigger big benefits for your body, including firing up your metabolism, adding lean muscle mass, and improving your aerobic and anaerobic capacity. But all that pounding can also create inflammation in muscles and joints and increase overall stress in the body, which is why I don't recommend running on certain days of the week on the Protocol. But if you like to jog, doing so on Day Two, when your inflammation and cortisol levels are super low and your blood is highly oxygenated, can help your body absorb all the benefits of the sport without any of its disadvantages.

2. **Lift heavy weights.** Day Two is the body's chance in the seven-day cycle to make big physiological gains, since inflammation levels are low and the blood is so oxygenated. If you like to lift weights, your body will have an easier time building muscle mass today. And while heavy lifting can tax the immune system, your body can handle it on Day Two, when your immune cells aren't overworked fighting other battles.

3. **Experiment.** What makes Day Two an ideal day to challenge your mind—greater mental clarity, focus, and emotional

stability—also makes it a prime day to challenge your body. You're more likely to have a pleasurable experience if you do something today that requires new movements or muscle coordination, like taking a dance class, signing up for a challenging yoga workshop, or trying a sport outside your comfort zone, like rock climbing, mountain biking, or tennis if you've never played. Since you're less prone to muscle pain and joint stiffness, any kind of new activity or movement you do today will also be less likely to leave you sore or creaky tomorrow.

Supplements: Best Nutrients to Take to Support Your Body and Mind Today

When you take your supplements, visualize them feeding the seeds you planted yesterday. Imagine that those seeds are beginning to sprout strong and healthy root systems throughout your body.

- Turmeric
- Wheatgrass
- Probiotics
- Royal jelly
- Lemon balm

Those with thyroid issues can take the following supplements in the morning, according to package instructions:

- Vitamin B_{12}
- Cat's claw
- Methylfolate

Those experiencing menopausal or perimenopausal symptoms can take the following supplements in the morning, according to package instructions:

- Red raspberry leaf extract
- Methylfolate

Those with depression or anxiety can take the following supplements in the morning, according to package instructions:

- Vitamin B_{12}

Those who have a viral infection (acute or chronic) can take the following supplements in the morning, according to package instructions:

- Lysine
- Cat's claw

Diet: Best Foods to Prioritize Today

Day Two gives you the opportunity to lower your inflammatory baseline—the level at which your body starts to build inflammation—and what you eat is one of the best ways to accomplish this goal. Today is not the time to load up on sugar, refined carbs, and other proinflammatory junk. Instead, focus on foods that will drive down inflammation, including the following seven foods, all of which have been shown by research to have a powerful anti-inflammatory effect in the brain and body:

- Broccoli
- Green tea
- Reishi mushrooms
- Lion's mane mushrooms
- Grapes
- Dark chocolate (prioritize dark and organic to minimize dairy—look for vegan alternatives high in beneficial cacao if you have a daily sensitivity or allergy)
- Dark cherries

DAY THREE: RESTORE

CHAPTER 9

The body's seven-day inflammation-detoxification cycle is very much like weathering a storm. Day Seven is the big event, Day One is the calm after the storm, Day Two is when everyone comes out to see the sunshine, and on Day Three, we begin to see the windows, shingles, trees, flowers, and all the other areas of our homes and yards that now need some love and attention.

To me, Day Three is the ultimate reset. Your body purged everything on Day Seven, recovered on Day One, went back to baseline on Day Two, and now on Day Three, you're finding your sense of equilibrium. When I think about the body today, I picture a set of balancing scales: The pans are parallel, and nothing is causing one side to tip lower than the other. In this sense, Day Three is similar to Day Two, when your body went back to baseline. Remember that the days of the Protocol are seamless—nothing immediately changes at midnight from one day to the next—and the characteristics of one day can flow into the following. In fact, the body flows through its circaseptan rhythms much like water moving down a river to exit into the ocean.

But there are also some big differences between Day Two and Day Three. While not much was going on biologically on Day Two, today your body is beginning to work on actively restocking and restoring itself. Essentially, your body is identifying any chinks it its armor and trying to plug those holes before it begins the rebuilding process on Day Four. This means your body is assessing what all your organs, muscles, and other tissues might need—for example, whether your liver requires a nutritional resupply, whether your stomach needs more material to manufacture digestive enzymes, and how your gallbladder is holding up. It's as though your body is looking at a big switchboard of all your body parts to see which areas may be lighting up, then answering the call and transferring nutrition where you need it. This is why eating foods rich in nutrients is so important on Day Three, as we'll detail at the end of this chapter.

Day Three can also be an empowering time for your body and mind. Like Day Two, you should feel physically, mentally, and emotionally stable today. But now, you may have even more energy, as your body actively works on resupplying itself, allowing you to make major gains in your healing, health, and life pursuits as you continue to follow the Protocol.

Biology: What Happens in Your Body Today

Day Three is when your cells mobilize. Your body ramps up production of stem cells today, which are the raw material from which specialized cells are made. Stem cells can also grow into new tissue, helping repair the body.

With stem cell production in a frenzy, your body also activates its stores of new red blood cells, which carry oxygen to organs and other tissue, along with new white blood cells, your body's immune cells that repair tissue, target foreign invaders, and help fight off illness. Overall, your circulatory system is extremely active today, as blood flow increases and more oxygen and nutrients are delivered throughout your body, especially to organs, muscles, and tissues that need it the most. Your blood pressure is likely more stable today than it is other days of the week; if you have hypertension, for instance, consider Day Three to be a little bit of a reprieve from all that fluid force on your arterial walls. Good blood pressure and increased circulation also help fortify the walls of your arteries and veins today, turning your vessels into superhighways that help transport nutrients more quickly and easily anywhere they need to go.

Helping this nutrient transport today is that your blood is especially alkaline, meaning it's less acidic, with a slightly higher pH. Otherwise, when your blood is acidic, your body can steal minerals like calcium and magnesium from healthy cells and organs in order to try to neutralize your blood.[1] This isn't a good thing since your cells need calcium and magnesium for hundreds of biological functions in the body, including building bone, relaxing muscle tissue, and regulating blood sugar. Acidic blood also increases the risk of disease, especially cancer, osteoporosis, and kidney disease.[2] Thankfully, that's not happening today, as your body uses its higher alkalinity to better support your metabolism, digestive system, and immune function.

Not only is your body producing more white blood cells today but it also has an entire fleet of T cells on standby, as they were on Day Two. Your body uses these T cells, which attack and destroy disease in the body, on Day Three to target any existing or chronic illness rather than try to mitigate inflammation, which is low today.

As your body identifies which areas need the most support today, it signals its stem cells to turn into specialized cells that can rebuild those areas on Day Four. The liver gets busy breaking down fat today to supply your body with essential lipids, which is particularly beneficial for your brain, along with your skin, hair, and nails. For this reason, Day Three is the best time of the week to indulge in a fatty meal if you must do it, since the body can digest these fats and put them to good use more readily than it can on other days of the week.

In short, Day Three is when your body is working to make sure it's entirely filled up and balanced, identifying and resupplying areas that need oxygen, nutrients, specialized cells, and other forms of physiological love.

Emotions: What Happens in Your Mind Today

You will likely feel more relaxed today, with enough calm energy to target and accomplish what you want to, thanks to improved blood pressure and blood flow. You might also be more receptive to new ideas or change. That's because when things are at an equilibrium internally, you're more open to novelty or even instability in external areas of your life.

Day Two was all about mental and emotional clarity, and this lucidity continues today—and it may feel slightly different. Instead of a simple presence of mind, you may feel more organized today, since you've had time to open your mind and receive new thoughts. If Day Two is when we gain new mental insight, Day Three is when we turn that insight into action.

You may also feel a sense of excitement today as your body starts to kick into gear and resupply and repair itself. This is very similar to a few days after a big storm, when the seas are tabletop calm, the skies have been bright for some time, and everyone is ready for action at last.

Daily Mantra: What to Tell Yourself to Stay Centered and Help Heal

To drive home today's purpose, give yourself permission to make your health and healing your top priority. Repeat today's mantra when you wake up and whenever you feel uncentered or uncertain throughout the day:

As my body repairs, I forgive myself and allow healing to take place.

Actions: Best Things to Do Today

1. **Focus on strategic thinking.** Our brains are made up of 60 percent fat and require a continual supply of fatty acids in order to fuel proper cognitive function. Without a doubt, your brain is getting those fatty acids today, as the liver breaks down fat and sends it throughout your body. That makes Day Three a prime opportunity to strategize in your professional or personal life, whether you need to brainstorm new ideas at work or develop an attack plan to accomplish your goals.

2. **Identify areas of your life that may need a little more love.** When you mirror what's happening inside you with what you do in your external world, you create a synergy between your body and life that can help you accomplish more. On Day Three, your body is identifying areas that need more nutrition and speeding nutrients there. Use this opportunity to figure out which relationships, projects, or behaviors may need your attention, addressing or starting to address what you can today.

3. **Attack any chores or tasks that you've been putting off.** Capitalize on your body's high-nutrient levels, low inflammation, and organizational clarity today to address those items on your to-do list that may have been sitting there a tad too long. You'll likely have more energy and eagerness to get things done, and you won't have as high a risk of depleting yourself as you do on other days of the week when your body is more inflamed or fatigued.

HEALTH: MEDICAL TESTS, TREATMENTS, AND THERAPIES TO PRIORITIZE TODAY

1. **Get your blood pressure checked.** Every medical professional knows that the body's blood pressure follows a circadian (twenty-four-hour) rhythm, rising in the morning when we

first get up, peaking in the afternoon, and falling in the evening before dropping even lower while we sleep. Similarly, our blood pressure has a circaseptan rhythm, too, peaking on Day Seven, falling on Day One, and rising again over the course of the week. On Day Three, the body's blood pressure is perfectly level, meaning it won't be inordinately higher due to your seven-day cycle. If you've had erratic blood pressure readings in the past or struggle with circulatory issues, try getting your blood pressure checked today–this will give you the most accurate reading of your base level. Be sure your doctor or nurse takes a reading in both arms to increase overall accuracy.

2. **Schedule any procedures that involve your circulatory system.** On Day Three, the body's circulatory system is very active, fortifying arterial walls and healing your entire vascular system. This makes today ideal for any interventions that involve the arteries, veins, or capillaries, including procedures like blood transfusions, intravenous surgery, stent or catheter placements, and varicose vein treatments. Not only will any intervention be less traumatic due to your lower inflammation levels and stable blood pressure but your circulatory system will also be able to heal more quickly, thanks to its increased nutrition.

3. **Opt for interventions that use extreme temperatures.** If you have to have an intervention that involves extreme heat or cold, like cryotherapy or cauterization, which are used to freeze or burn abnormal cells or tissue, respectively, schedule that procedure for Day Three. Since the body's blood is especially alkaline today, extreme temps won't shock your system as much–otherwise, the exposure, especially to cold temps, can cause your blood to become more acidic,[3] increasing your risk of illness and disease.

---

1. **Try cryotherapy or take an ice bath.** When used strategically as part of your self-care regimen, extreme cold can boost your body's ability to heal. That's because exposing yourself to really cold temperatures activates molecules known as heat-shock proteins (HSPs), which identify and repair damaged proteins, helping to reduce inflammation,[4] mend muscle tissue,[5] and even help treat some autoimmune disease.[6] While it's best not to sit in an ice bath Days Five through One-the extreme temps can add stress to your system and affect your blood pH-you'll be able to reap all the benefits of cryotherapy, or cold therapy, on Day Three.

   Cryotherapy has been used to ease chronic pain, treat cancer, and trigger hormonal changes that may mitigate mood disorders like anxiety and depression, according to studies.[7] Some spas, physical therapy clinics, integrative-medicine clinics, and gyms offer cryotherapy services, where you can sit in a temperature-controlled machine for a specific period of time. The sessions can be pricey, however, so if you don't have the money or can't find a cryotherapy service nearby, you can create the experience at home by taking an ice bath and soaking for no more than ten minutes.

2. **Take an infrared sauna, steam bath, hot yoga class, or soak in a hot tub.** As with cryotherapy, exposing yourself to really hot temps today also increases healing without placing undue stress on the body when it may not be able to handle it. My favorite form of heat therapy is an infrared sauna, which uses special lamps to heat your body directly rather than heating the air around you like traditional saunas do. Like cryotherapy, infrared saunas also activate HSPs and have been shown by research to treat chronic pain, ease chronic fatigue syndrome, stimulate weight loss, and boost heart health.[8] If you choose to take an infrared sauna, talk

with your doctor first, since some health conditions like low blood pressure and kidney disease can make intense heat dangerous, and limit your sessions to no more than twenty minutes.[9] Exposing yourself to sustained heat today, whether you sit in a sauna, steam bath, or hot tub, or take a hot yoga class, will also dilate your blood vessels, helping speed nutrient delivery to all your organs, muscles, and tissues.

3. **Experiment with oil pulling.** The ancient Ayurvedic practice of oil pulling is super easy to do—and can have big benefits on Day Three. To oil pull, you simply swish cold-pressed virgin coconut oil in your mouth for fifteen to twenty minutes before spitting it out. This, in turn, helps increase internal alkalinity by removing toxins and excess acids from the mouth.[10] While your blood is already more alkaline on Day Three, alkalizing it further can help establish a new baseline you can retain for the rest of the week and even into the following week. And the more alkaline your blood, the lower your risk of inflammation and disease.

Brett's Story: The Power of Day Three

Imagine that you're one of the most successful players in the NFL, at the top of your career and having a phenomenal season, when you tear your ACL—not once but twice. That's what happened to one player when we started working together again several years ago. I had known Brett through one of his fellow teammates, and while he knew something about the Protocol, he hadn't been following it. But after his second ACL tear and second subsequent surgery, he called me in a panic. Brett's range of motion was destroyed, he had only a fraction of his former strength, and he was worried he would lose his contract. He was also in a lot of pain and fisting a ton of painkillers to be able to make it through his workouts.

When we tested his blood, I wasn't surprised to see that Brett's inflammatory markers were through the roof. I immediately put him on the Protocol, making sure he took the right supplements at the right time to bring down inflammation in his knee, as well as throughout his entire body. I also worked with the rest of his medical team to reduce the dosage of painkillers he was taking, which were masking his pain, not improving it, and allowing him to push through workouts when he shouldn't.

As a pro player, Brett had access to cryotherapy and hot saunas whenever he wanted, but I told him he should use these only on Days Two through Four—and especially on Day Three. This way, he'd get all the benefits of heat-shock proteins when we knew his system could handle the additional stress and not turn his blood acidic.

I also recommended that Brett do demanding workouts only on Day Three. Before I started working with him, his routine involved lifting heavy weights, running in a hyperbaric chamber, and doing drills with sleds and pop-up tacklers whenever he scheduled time with his physical-therapy team. But all that taxing exercise, when done on the wrong days of the week, was actually impeding his ability to heal and get stronger: When he did these workouts on Days Five, Six, Seven, or One, he was just adding inflammation to existing inflammation. I convinced him that if he could reschedule these intense workouts to Day Three, when his blood was speeding more oxygen and nutrients to his muscles, joints, and ligaments, he would make faster strength gains and improve his recovery time.

After just two weeks on the Protocol, in addition to using Day Three for hard workouts, cryotherapy, and sauna treatments, Brett was able to increase how much weight he was able to lift with his injured leg. His range of motion improved and his pain subsided. At this point, we were able to get him off the painkillers. After the painkillers had cleared his blood, we ran his lab work again, which showed his inflammatory markers were under control: His body could finally heal.

Six months later, Brett was off the injured list and back on the starting lineup. He's been able to make a full recovery since then—and he now tells me he'll live by the Protocol as often as he can, viewing it as his biggest safety net to help prevent another career-threatening injury.

EXERCISE: BEST WAYS TO MOVE YOUR BODY TODAY

1. **Do high-intensity interval training.** With more blood, oxygen, and nutrients flowing freely to muscles, Day Three is ideal for high-intensity interval training (HIIT). HIIT alternates

short, intense bursts of cardio–think sprinting, stair climbing, jumping rope, and plyometric drills–with periods of active recovery. The workouts are challenging, but the rewards are a faster metabolism, increased calorie burn, quicker weight loss, better muscle gain, lower blood pressure, and improved blood sugar regulation.[11] While these benefits are impressive, it's important to be strategic about when you're doing HIIT: Prioritize your superhard workouts on Days Two through Four to get your biggest gains and fastest recovery.

2. **Do a race, take a fitness test, or otherwise push your body to perform.** For the same reasons that make HIIT ideal for Day Three, competing in a race, fitness test, or other high-performance physical event is also befitting for today. Not only will you be able to go harder and longer but you'll also recover more quickly.

3. **Go for a long bike ride, hike, run, or row.** If you enjoy endurance exercise, Day Three is the time to do it. With your liver busy breaking down fat, your body can more easily and effectively tap into that fuel supply to sustain distance workouts today. You'll also wake up less sore tomorrow, since you have less inflammation and increased blood and nutrient flow than on other days of the week.

Supplements: Best Nutrients to Take to Support Your Body and Mind Today

When you take your supplements, visualize that you're helping the root system of your body push up strong stalks that will now begin to reach for the sunlight.

- Turmeric
- Wheatgrass
- Probiotics
- Royal jelly
- Lemon balm

Those with thyroid issues can take the following supplements in the morning, according to package instructions:

- Vitamin B_{12}
- Cat's claw
- Methylfolate

Those experiencing menopausal or perimenopausal symptoms can take the following supplements in the morning, according to package instructions:

- Red raspberry leaf extract
- Methylfolate

Those with depression or anxiety can take the following supplements in the morning, according to package instructions:

- Vitamin B_{12}

Those who have a viral infection (acute or chronic) can take the following supplements in the morning, according to package instructions:

- Lysine
- Cat's claw

Diet: Best Foods to Prioritize Today

Today is the time to maximize your micronutrient intake in order to enrich your blood with what it needs to deliver vitamins, minerals, and antioxidants to organs and other tissues. Additionally, Day Three is a good day to eat foods that improve alkalinity. While your blood is already alkaline, prioritizing foods that increase blood pH can help you establish a new baseline for your body for the rest of the week. Alkaline foods counter the inflammatory effects of acidic foods like meat, dairy, added sugar, processed foods, and many other items the average American eats every day. Some alkalizing foods like citrus fruits may contain acid, but they don't have an acidic effect in the body—quite the opposite: lemons, oranges, and grapefruits help alkalize blood. In addition to those, try the following:

- Almonds
- Spinach
- Parsley
- Avocados
- Red onions
- Basil

DAY FOUR: REBUILD

CHAPTER 10

O ne thing I love about the Protocol is that it gives you the chance to celebrate every day for no other reason than what's happening in your body. And on Day Four, what's happening in your body is really, really special. Today is when your body rebuilds.

While this may sound like a lot of work, it's not laborious for your body. Instead, Day Four is all about self-love, as you take the time to restore and refresh your muscles, bones, organs, and other tissues. After receiving so much oxygen and nutrition on Day Three, you're on cloud nine right now, with the same sense of satisfaction you might feel after sharing a really good meal with friends. In other words, Day Four is delicious.

Today, all your muscles, bones, connective tissue, and organs are beginning to put the nutrients they received yesterday to work, actively rebuilding tissue, repairing muscle, fortifying bone, and preventing scar tissue before it can form. When I think about Day Four, the words *regeneration, reinvigoration, reawaken,* and *re-creation* come to mind.

There's also a certain sense of luxury today, since you're giving your body what it needs. It's like your body is having a birthday, and all its parts are being showered with a million tiny gifts. You feel satisfied and whole, which is why Day Four is often the best day of the week for many people, when they tell me they feel their happiest or most content.

Every day is a gift, but Day Four can feel like a particular largesse. Be sure to take advantage of it and let the joy in, body, mind, and spirit.

Biology: What Happens in Your Body Today

On Day Three, your body was busy making new stem cells—the most basic cells in the human body from which almost all other cells form. Now, on Day Four, those stem cells are turning into specialized cells, including satellite cells, which work to help repair muscle. You don't have to be an athlete to benefit from this muscular mending: Everyone incurs wear and tear and muscular inflammation, even those who never see the inside of a gym or do anything active all week. In fact, too much sitting can increase muscle inflammation,[1] so if you're a desk jockey, you'll benefit big-time from Day Four.

One of the biggest muscles to rebuild on Day Four is your heart, as satellite cells start to regenerate damaged tissue in the body's hardest working muscle. You can have a very healthy heart and still have damaged tissue, too—tissue damage is a natural occurrence on Days Six and Seven as the body goes through its seven-day inflammation-detoxification cycle.

On Day Four, our stem cells also turn into osteoblasts—cells that help build new bone—and fibroblasts, which repair tendons, ligaments, and fascia. This creates a strong synergy throughout your musculoskeletal system, as muscles, bones, and connective tissue work together to refortify and restrengthen. Day Four is an incredibly powerful time for all the structural parts that support the body.

We already know the liver gets taxed on Days Six and Seven, when it has to process, break down, and metabolize a seven-day buildup of hormones, cellular waste, toxins, and other inflammatory markers. But on Day Four, your liver is taking an opportunity to heal itself, using the nutrients it received on Day Three to regenerate cells damaged during the detoxification process. The same goes for your digestive tract, which replaces and restores the epithelium, or the cells that line the stomach and intestines. This also boosts the health of your immune system, 70 percent of which is found in the gut.[2]

One of the most amazing things about Day Four? It's your body's best chance to beautify. The body heals from the inside out, so it will always prioritize your internal organs, muscles, and bones first. But after your body directs its cellular support, nutrients, and energy to rebuilding your internal parts, it will focus on its external areas, primarily your skin, hair, and nails. If you actively work to improve your health by eating right and living by the Protocol, you'll reduce your inflammation and overall toxic load, boosting your body's ability to better support your skin, hair, and nails.

Emotions: What Happens in Your Mind Today

Day Four is when most people tell me that they feel their best. This includes my patients with life-threatening illnesses: They're almost always calmer, more relaxed, more easygoing, and more amenable to changes in their treatment or even hearing bad news. But no matter how sick or perfectly healthy they are, most patients tell me they feel more fulfillment or satisfaction on Day Four. And whenever I see them in person, they're often glowing with good health, which radiates from the inside out.

You can expect to feel more content, whole, and satisfied on Day Four, too. The mental and emotional clarity you enjoyed on Days Two and Three often turns into gratification. Even if everything isn't right with your health or professional or personal life, you may feel more laid-back today, more willing to go with the flow, more able to accept or even embrace change, and even more willing to tolerate things as they are.

I like to use Day Four to practice self-love and gratitude. From a biological perspective, these feelings are easier to manifest today, but it's up to you to consciously tap into and bring them to the surface. If you do, you can use this gratitude as a powerful antidote, since I believe that feeling grateful can improve your physical and mental health as much as any prescription drug or medical intervention.

Of course, it's possible to feel negative today, especially if external factors come up that you have no control over. At the same time, your body is set up to feel really good, so if you do get bad news or something unfortunate occurs, consider it a gift that this negative energy is trying to unseat you on the day when you are biologically and psychologically best equipped to let it roll off your back.

Daily Mantra: What to Tell Yourself to Stay Centered and Help Heal

To drive home today's purpose, empower yourself by honoring your life, your path, and your body. Repeat the following mantra when you wake up and whenever you feel uncentered or uncertain throughout the day:

I have the power to rebuild my life, my emotions, and my body.

Actions: Best Things to Do Today

1. Be social. Capitalize on your feelings of contentment, wholeness, and self-love today by letting your light shine through with others. Day Four is a great time to get together with friends, host a dinner party, meet new people, or go on a date. Whether you're single, in a relationship, or married, you may also be more attractive to others today, since you're coming from a place of wholeness and empowerment.

2. Take a trip down memory lane. Since everything in your body is level and complete today, you'll be more apt to look back fondly on old memories rather than view the past with anger, resentment, or regret. I always tell patients that Day Four is the ideal time to work on a family photo album, reconnect with old acquaintances, or bring up issues from your past that you want to work through with others.

3. Make a high-risk decision. If you want to ask for a raise, quit your job, make a large purchase, pop the question to your significant other—or make any other decision that could have significant or lasting ramifications—today is the day to do it. Not only are you super emotionally and mentally stable today but your body isn't taxed. You're enjoying the most strategic mindset you will have all week, which allows you to make important choices for the right reasons.

HEALTH: MEDICAL TESTS, TREATMENTS, AND THERAPIES TO PRIORITIZE TODAY

1. See a chiropractor or osteopath. Your skeletal system is in full rebuild mode, so if you see a chiropractor or osteopath (doctors who specifically treat the entire musculoskeletal system) today, your bones will be more pliable to any adjustments, helping realignment last longer. Spinal adjustments in general also trigger the production of more bone-building osteoblasts, which, on Day Four, your body will be able to utilize immediately.

2. **Get deep-tissue work.** Like your bones, your muscles are also busy rebuilding today, more so than on any other day of the week. Similar to receiving spinal adjustments, if you have any deep-tissue work done today, whether it's deep-tissue massage, Rolfing, or fascial scraping, it will stimulate new cell formation that your body can more readily incorporate into your muscles today. You'll also recover more quickly from intense muscular manipulation today since the body's inflammation levels are lower and your muscles, tendons, ligaments, and fascia are all rich with nutrition.

3. **Schedule spinal or orthopedic surgery.** If you have to have surgery for a herniated disk, torn ACL, broken bone, or other spinal, tendon, or soft-tissue injury, schedule it for Day Four. Oftentimes, these kinds of operations are an emergency—in which case you should have the procedure as soon as possible. But if it isn't urgent and you have a choice in the matter, opting to have spinal or orthopedic operations on Day Four will increase the efficacy and success of surgery while reducing your recovery time.

SELF-CARE: BEST WAYS TO NOURISH YOUR BODY, MIND, AND SPIRIT TODAY

1. **Get acupuncture.** Since your body is restacking and rebuilding today, it's more receptive to establishing new patterns and pathways. This means if you receive acupuncture on Day Four, it has a greater chance of creating or restoring healthy energy flow throughout your meridians. This energy flow also has a higher likelihood of lasting for a longer period of time when you receive acupuncture on Day Four on a regular basis, since the body gets used to rebuilding the same way in our seven-day cycle.

2. **Go for a manicure or pedicure.** While they may look lovely, manicures and pedicures can cause a ton of microtrauma to nails. Filing, cutting, and using toxic polish removers and paints can take a toll on our nail beds, cuticles, and surrounding skin when done regularly enough. Minimize that damage by opting to get a mani or pedi on Day Four only, when your nails can best withstand and rebuild from the trauma.

3. **Schedule skin treatment.** Day Four is ideal for exfoliation, microneedling, or similar skin treatment. That's because our skin is rich with nutrients, low in inflammation, and most receptive to the end goal of any facial procedure.

EXERCISE: BEST WAYS TO MOVE YOUR BODY TODAY

1. **Try power lifting.** If you like to lift really heavy weights, today is the day to do it. Since power lifting tears down muscles—sometimes to the point where you do more harm than good—you want to be discerning about which days you inflict that kind of trauma on your body. On Day Four, however, you'll recover more quickly from muscle breakdown and actually be better able to rebuild, which is the whole end goal of the exercise.

2. **Do Pilates, ballet, or other exercises that lengthen muscle.** Since your muscles are more elastic and pliable today, you'll likely feel good doing exercises that lengthen muscle tissue, like Pilates and ballet. What's more, focusing on stretching and extending can have greater benefits today than other days of the week. That's because your body is rebuilding and restructuring, thereby enabling it to incorporate any new length you create into its framework.

3. **Play tackle football or take a boxing or kickboxing class.** If you're going to sustain a hard hit to your muscles, bones, and connective tissue, today is the day you'll want to do it, since

your body will be able to repair and recover more quickly from the trauma.

Ashley's Story: The Power of Day Four

When most people hear the word *muscles*, they think abs, quadriceps, biceps, glutes, and all the other tissue we use to play sports and want to tone before a big date or beach vacation. But muscles are also found in surprising areas of the body like the stomach and play a critical role in our physiological function.

Muscles make up our gastrointestinal tract and are necessary to move food through the gut. But if they lose tone—which can happen due to too much stress, inflammation, a bacterial imbalance, or nutritional deficiencies[3]—what we eat gets backed up in the GI tract, causing undigested particles and toxins to seep into the bloodstream. The condition, known as gastroparesis, can interfere with immune health, since undigested foods can sit in the gut so long that it starts to change the balance of healthy bacteria in our microbiome, which influences our immunity.

There's something else I see all the time in patients who lose stomach muscle tone: They get diagnosed with a food sensitivity they don't have. Gastroparesis can cause the body to start manufacturing antibodies to undigested food particles—not because people are sensitive to a food but because they're not digesting that particular food due to lack of muscle tone. When patients get diagnosed with a food sensitivity, suddenly they cut out all these foods or adopt an extremely restrictive diet, which only aggravates their condition.

This was exactly what was happening when Ashley and I started working together several years ago. The thirty-six-year-old came to see me because she couldn't regulate her digestion: She was either constipated or had diarrhea—there was no middle ground—and her stomach was always bloated and distended. She'd been diagnosed with a number of food sensitivities, including to soy, corn, dairy, eggs, and sulfites, all of which she subsequently removed from her diet. She'd also cut out a number of foods on her own accord because she believed they'd either leave her with diarrhea for days or make her constipated. By the time we met, Ashely had severe disordered eating, triggered by a fear of feeling sick, and she was eating only oyster crackers and drinking Diet Coke. This had only worsened her health problems, as you can imagine, and she developed a thyroid disorder, chronic dermatitis, and dry, brittle hair, despite her best efforts to exercise and otherwise live a healthy life.

The first thing I did, of course, was get Ashely on the Protocol. But her body was so malnourished that we had more to do than simply sync her life with her seven-day cycle. When I looked through her health records, I saw she had been tested for food sensitivities on Day Six—one of the worst days possible, since inflammation and histamine (chemicals produced in response to allergens) levels are so high, which can interfere with a test's accuracy. I convinced Ashley to get retested on Day Four when her body's natural markers were lower, and her stomach lining would be healthier.

Perhaps the biggest advantage to testing on Day Four would be that the muscles in her GI tract would be working as optimally as they could, having just received a full resupply of nutrients, including the minerals magnesium, which helps calm muscles, and calcium, which helps muscles contract.

After Ashley was retested, we discovered that she really didn't have sensitivities to all the foods she thought she did—her results only showed a dairy sensitivity. But this didn't explain why she was still experiencing crippling symptoms, which were very real. So what was causing all of Ashley's bloating, diarrhea, and constipation?

Because she had adopted such a restrictive diet, Ashley wasn't getting the magnesium, calcium, and other nutrients she needed to build and preserve muscle tone in her stomach, which, in turn, had triggered a case of gastroparesis. Ashley needed to start eating a wider variety of foods, but given her history and mindset—she truly believed eating almost anything other than bland carbs would make her sick—I knew we had to progress slowly.

For the same reasons that Day Four is ideal for food-sensitivity testing, it's also the best day to reintroduce items back into your diet. We started Ashely out slowly, having her consume one new food every two weeks until she was eating grain-free breads, beans, eggs, and whole vegetables and fruit. After several months, her hair started to grow again, the dermatitis went away, and her thyroid levels reregulated. As she continued to live by the Protocol and properly nourish her GI tract, her constipation, diarrhea, and bloating eventually disappeared.

Today, Ashley is still slightly paranoid around food—a byproduct of years of disordered eating and illness. But her symptoms are completely gone, and she's a much happier, healthier person than she says she ever imagined she could be.

Supplements: Best Nutrients to Take
to Support Your Body and Mind Today

When you take your supplements, visualize the stalk you've nurtured over the last several days now climbing higher and higher, reaching toward the sun and beginning to form a healthy, hearty bud.

- Turmeric
- Wheatgrass
- Probiotics
- Royal jelly
- Lemon balm

Those with thyroid issues can take the following supplements in the morning, according to package instructions:

- Vitamin B_{12}
- Cat's claw
- Methylfolate

Those experiencing menopausal or perimenopausal symptoms can take the following supplements in the morning, according to package instructions:

- Red raspberry leaf extract
- Methylfolate

Those with depression or anxiety can take the following supplements in the morning, according to package instructions:

- Vitamin B_{12}

Those who have a viral infection (acute or chronic) can take the following supplements in the morning, according to package instructions:

- Lysine
- Cat's claw

Diet: Best Foods to Prioritize Today

Your body needs a maximum amount of protein today in order to help repair and rebuild muscle. You'll also want to make sure you're getting all essential amino acids, with items like eggs, salmon, and sunflower seeds. Finally, you'll want to prioritize antioxidant-rich foods like the ones listed here as much as possible to help your liver regenerate and your muscles, bones, and organs build the healthiest tissue possible.

- Arugula
- Eggs
- Salmon
- Blueberries
- Sunflower seeds
- Cauliflower
- Sweet potatoes

DAY FIVE: PREPARATION

CHAPTER 11

Day Five is the last of the halcyon days. After today, your body enters the second stage of the Protocol, Days Six and Seven, when it instigates a whirlwind of inflammation and detoxification. Your seven-day cycle moves toward this crescendo all week, and on Day Five, there's an awareness that your body is about to go into turmoil. This makes Day Five the calm before the storm, the time when your body prepares for what's about to happen by boarding up its windows and battening down the hatches.

For these reasons, your body is a little weaker today, just like it was on Day One when recovering from its weekly inflammation-detoxification cycle. Today, however, you're slightly more sensitive, as your body anticipates and prepares— physically, emotionally, and spiritually—for what's about to take place tomorrow and the next day. Biologically, this manifests as an uptick in activity in your kidneys and liver toward the end of Day Five, as your body begins to produce more hormones that, in excess, cause inflammation.

While all this is happening, you can still expect to feel pretty energetic on Day Five. Your internal organs, musculoskeletal system, and immune system have all been bathed in nutrition and built back up again, and your blood is still happily alkaline. Despite increasing slightly by the end of the day, your hormones are relatively stable, and your other inflammatory markers are comparatively low.

That's all good news, as you'll want to try to harness all the mental clarity and positive energy you can today. Day Five is the best day of the week to reflect on and reevaluate your goals. You've just had five consecutive days of stability and progression, so you're in a good place to analyze your success so far and which areas may need improvement.

Biology: What Happens in Your Body Today

On Day Five, your body goes on alert. Pain receptors, which are nerve cells that detect damage or the threat of damage, start to become more responsive today, activating your central nervous system. Your immune system also begins to ramp up, galvanizing its gang of T cells to attack any foreign invaders in your body. Your in-house army of more than ten million antibodies is also more active today, as it works to identify which markers in the body are foreign and which are simply part of your seven-day cycle.

For the most part, your liver is on cruise control today, although it does start to produce more bile. Bile helps the body digest fats and eliminate old red blood cells and toxins—a key preparatory step before your body begins to detoxify, like filling up a car's gas tank before a big road trip. For some people, this extra bile can cause indigestion and acid reflux.

One of the more exciting things to take place today is that your skin cells regenerate. This occurs every week until your entire epidermis—the outside layer of skin—is replaced, which happens every three weeks. This weekly regeneration makes Day Five your biggest and best opportunity to heal wounds and other forms of skin damage. While Day Four is still the best day for facials and other cosmetic treatments, know that your body is actively healing—visualize this if skin damage is a concern for you.

Lots of things are happening in your heart today, too. After the increased alkalinity and nutrient and oxygen flow, low blood pressure, and muscle rebuilding of Days Three and Four, your heart is stronger than ever, with improved muscle tone and circulation.

Toward the end of the day, both your kidney and liver function begin to increase. As we've already discussed, your liver starts producing more bile while your kidneys start to discharge more protein and mineral salts, both of which are detectable in urine—why your pee may look a little cloudier today. At the end of the day, inflammatory markers like C-reactive protein, uric acid, and cortisol, along with testosterone and estrogen, begin to increase.

Emotions: What Happens in Your Mind Today

You can expect to still feel pretty good today in terms of your energy and focus. At the same time, you may notice that you are becoming a little more sensitive or aware of what's happening around you. This can cause some people to be touchy or testy today, increasing the likelihood that you may perceive what other people say or do as possible slights against you—something to be aware of as you navigate the day.

Some of my patients also tell me that they feel a little anxious on Day Five, as though they are packing for a trip and keep wondering whether they've forgotten something. If you feel more tense, take a breath and remember that your body is anticipating and preparing for what's right around the corner. It's a natural process and not something to cause you worry or angst.

On the plus side, Day Five is when most of my new patients report feeling the first positive effects of the Protocol. It makes sense, too: You've enjoyed five straight days of aligning your body with its natural seven-day cycle, in addition to taking powerful anti-inflammatory supplements. These initial positive effects are unique to each person, but in general, many of my patients tell me they notice increased energy, improved weight loss, better focus, and more mental clarity after five days on the Protocol.

Daily Mantra: What to Tell Yourself to Stay Centered and Help Heal

To drive home today's purpose, recognize that change isn't frightening: It signifies great growth and transformation. Repeat the following mantra when you wake up and whenever you feel uncentered or uncertain throughout the day:

I will find strength in change.

Actions: Best Things to Do Today

1. **Take care of loose ends.** *Don't put off until tomorrow what you can do today* is an extremely apt proverb for Day Five. Since you're likely to feel a little lethargic tomorrow and the next day, today is a good opportunity to attack anything you want to do with gusto, including knocking off your to-do list, working through your emails, or doing any shopping or cleaning that can't wait. Think of it like getting ready for a big storm: There's a possibility you could be out of commission for two days, so try to make the most of what you're able to accomplish today.

2. **Don't rock the boat.** Day Five may not be your big time to shine and confront your boss, have a potentially inflammatory conversation with a family member, or make a momentous decision that could leave you otherwise feeling vulnerable. You're sensitive today, and if you rock the boat in any way, you're more likely to feel like you're falling overboard. What's more, if you have big conversations or make any momentous decisions today that cause ripple effects into tomorrow or the next day, you won't be well suited to handle those ramifications. Instead, use this day to prepare for anything you need to do, not only over the next two days but also the next week and beyond. Your body is in preparation mode, so take advantage of it!

3. **Go ahead and have a cheat meal or that extra drink.** If you're going to eat sugary, processed food or overindulge in cocktails, today is the day to do so. Since your body will start detoxifying tomorrow, you'll be able to more readily and quickly get rid of any sugar, booze, gluten, dairy, and other dietary toxins. But don't go overboard: Just because you're detoxifying the next two days doesn't mean you should consume all the pizza, ice cream, and wine you can get your hands on. Eating or drinking too many inflammatory substances can overwhelm your body and intensify illness and inflammation, along with feelings of fatigue, brain fog, anxiety, and depression.

HEALTH: MEDICAL TESTS, TREATMENTS, AND THERAPIES TO PRIORITIZE TODAY

1. **Opt for chemotherapy.** For the same reasons Day Five is ideal for a cheat meal, it's also a good time to schedule chemotherapy if you're undergoing cancer treatment. Chemotherapy is toxic—so much so that the drugs are dangerous for doctors to handle. While you want the treatment to kill cancer cells, you also don't want it to linger in your body so long that it kills a

lot of healthy cells, too. If you have a choice when to receive chemo, opt for Day Five if and when you can.

2. **Avoid dialysis and gastric procedures.** Today is one of the worst days for dialysis, which treats kidney malfunction or failure. The therapy, which removes excess waste and fluid from the blood, can also shock the kidneys, which are sensitive on Day Five. You'll also want to steer clear of stomach procedures: Excess bile produced by the liver can back up into the gastrointestinal tract, causing inflammation and other problems that could complicate a surgery or other interventions.

3. **Schedule any medical procedures that can't wait at least two days.** Advance warning: You're going to want to avoid most kinds of health care that aren't emergencies on Days Six and Seven. For this reason, Day Five is your last ideal day to undergo any nonurgent procedure. While certain medical interventions are better suited to Days Two, Three, or Four, as we've covered in preceding chapters, if the choice is between receiving medical care today or waiting until tomorrow, the next day, or even the morning of Day One, opt to receive that care today.

SELF-CARE: BEST WAYS TO NOURISH YOUR BODY, MIND, AND SPIRIT TODAY

1. **Schedule any self-care treatments that can't wait at least two days.** Similar to medical procedures, if there are any self-care treatments like acupuncture, lymphatic massage, cryotherapy, or Reiki that you'd like to do, schedule them on Dave Five–or wait at least two days before opting to have them.

2. **Focus on reflexology.** Reflexology is the practice of applying pressure to certain areas of the foot to influence the health and energy flow of organs and bodily systems that connect to

those areas. Studies show that targeted reflexology can boost blood flow to the kidneys—beneficial today, since these organs are starting to work harder—and help lower stress and anxiety.[1] Receiving reflexology on Day Five can also increase energy flow to other bodily systems, helping fortify them before they begin processing biotoxins.

3. **Set and observe boundaries.** If you feel particularly sensitive today, take the time to recognize and accept that feeling. To help better navigate this emotion, use today to set personal boundaries as soon as you wake up. You can choose to say no to other people's needs or drama or decide not to absorb unsolicited criticism. Whatever boundary you decide to set, make an intention to do so in the morning and try to stick with it throughout the day.

All about Lymphatic Massage

Day Five is ideal for lymphatic massage, also called manual lymphatic drainage, a form of light massage that encourages movement of lymph fluid. The practice can help the body reduce swelling and filter and eliminate more toxins. I recommend lymphatic massage to all my patients on Day Five, since the technique stimulates toxin flow to the liver before the organ undergoes the Cleanse, which will help your body better eliminate these toxins. Anyone with pronounced puffiness can also benefit from lymphatic massage, while it may also help reduce symptoms of rheumatoid arthritis, fibromyalgia, and several other conditions,[2] along with pain and inflammation associated with sports injuries.[3] If you're undergoing chemotherapy or radiation or have a serious medical condition, particularly congestive heart failure or problems with skin infection, check with your doctor before scheduling a massage with a certified practitioner.

EXERCISE: BEST WAYS TO
MOVE YOUR BODY TODAY

1. **Switch to low impact.** Days Two, Three, and Four are great for workouts that include running, interval training, heavy lifting, or other forms of intense or high-impact exercise. But on Day Five, your body switches its energy from resettling, restoring, and rebuilding to preparing. Complement that shift by prioritizing low-intensity and low-impact movement like swimming, yoga, and resistance-band training.

2. **Get your wiggles out, if you're that type.** While low-impact exercise is best for Day Five, if you're the type of person who feels more mentally or emotionally centered after a tough workout, it's better to go hard today than allow yourself to feel pent-up and decide to do a more challenging workout Day Six or Seven. Personally, I can't go three days in a row without a hard workout: Intense exercise is a mental and emotional outlet for me and form of moving meditation. If that sounds like you, go ahead and do something intense today, but try to switch the type of difficult workout or tempo from what you might do Days Two through Four. For example, if you usually power lift, try doing a hard run or vice versa—and don't overlook resistance bands, which can give you an intense workout all on their own. This is what I recommend to my patients who are professional athletes and don't have a choice about whether they take three consecutive days off from hard exercise.

3. **Walk and reflect.** One of the ways to move your body on Day Five is to take a long, low-impact walk—anywhere from twenty-five to ninety minutes, depending on what seems long for your usual routine. This way, you'll get your heart rate up, your metabolism moving, and your blood pumping, all of which will help fortify your body for processing toxins tomorrow and the next day. Taking a long walk can also give you the headspace you need to reflect on the progress you've made this week and what you may want to do differently or the same next week.

Finally, going for a long walk can help you prepare mentally for what's about to come.

Michael's Story: The Power of Day Five

The way our skin regenerates on Day Five is nothing short of miraculous. When I met Michael three months after his failed second surgery to put in a pacemaker, the forty-seven-year-old was in serious need of a miracle.

Michael has something called mitral valve prolapse, a condition that occurs when the valve that separates the upper and lower chambers of the left side of the heart doesn't close properly. In most people the condition is asymptomatic, but in Michael's case, the prolapse had caused his blood to flow backward into his heart, damaging the organ and leaving him with chest pain, fatigue, and shortness of breath. He needed a pacemaker to help regulate his heartbeat and prevent blood regurgitation, and when he was in his midthirties, he underwent surgery to have the device installed.

But less than a year later, Michael had developed a staph infection around the surgical wound, which had never fully healed. As a result, his body rejected the pacemaker, and his doctors told him he needed another operation to prevent the risk of congestive heart failure.

Several years later, Michael went under the knife again—this time at a different hospital with a different surgeon, which he hoped would improve his results. But the same thing happened: Within months, his wound was infected, and his doctors were delivering the same message as his original surgeon had. This was when he called me.

When we started working together, Michael's inflammation levels were through the roof, which was obvious in his blood work. I got him on the Protocol immediately, and he started to take the supplements recommended in chapter 4, also following the program's anti-inflammatory diet, swapping out his daily pizza and steak for more healing foods like grilled salmon, zucchini pasta, and sweet potato bean burritos. Per the Protocol, we worked to make sure he was also syncing his daily habits with his seven-day cycle, not overpowering what his body wanted to do the days it needed to rest and relax. At the same time, Michael started to incorporate more mindfulness into his day by meditating. All these steps helped slash his inflammation significantly when we retested several weeks later.

But Michael still needed a pacemaker, and while it was great that his inflammation levels were so much lower, I knew that we had to figure out a way to get his body to accept the device. I began to look at why his past surgeries had been unsuccessful. He had seen different surgeons at two different hospitals, making it unlikely that medical expertise or environment played a role in his wound problems. The only reason that was obvious to me was that Michael had undergone surgery both times on his Day Seven, which happened to be a Tuesday.

I told Michael to schedule his third operation for Sunday—his Day Five. While the day isn't ideal for invasive procedures, it's great for wound healing, which is what Michael's body needed the most. What's more, his heart would be strongest on Day Five, which would increase the likelihood that the cardiac procedure would be successful.

With a little legwork, Michael found a surgeon who was willing to operate over the weekend, and he underwent a third procedure to install a pacemaker. Six weeks later, with no signs of wound infection, his pain and fatigue began to recede for the first time in decades. That was five years ago. Today, he still has the same pacemaker, which his body fully accepted, and is now playing golf, walking, and enjoying exercise again.

Supplements: Best Nutrients to Take to Support Your Body and Mind Today

When you take your supplements, visualize your body's bud growing bigger and bigger as you feed it the nutrients it needs to bloom.

- Turmeric
- Wheatgrass
- Probiotics
- Royal jelly
- Lemon balm

Those with thyroid issues can take the following supplements in the morning, according to package instructions:

- Vitamin B_{12}
- Cat's claw
- Methylfolate

Those experiencing menopausal or perimenopausal symptoms can take the following supplements in the morning, according to package instructions:

- Red raspberry leaf extract
- Methylfolate

Those with depression or anxiety can take the following supplements in the morning, according to package instructions:

- Vitamin B_{12}

Those who have a viral infection (acute or chronic) can take the following supplements in the morning, according to package instructions:

- Lysine
- Cat's claw

Diet: Best Foods to Prioritize Today

Today's a great day to prioritize foods packed with antioxidants, which will help fuel optimal skin repair. Black beans, berries, and dark, leafy vegetables like collard greens top the list of foods with the most antioxidants per gram. Beans, edamame, and fresh veggies and fruit also boost cardiovascular health, helping your heart establish a new baseline as it beats stronger today than it will all week.

- Collard greens
- Kidney beans
- Black beans
- Edamame (organic only, to avoid genetically modified soy)
- Blackberries
- Raspberries

DAY SIX: FLUSH

CHAPTER 12

Them is is the chapter many of you have been waiting for—or, at the very least, are curious about. What happens when your body repeats the trauma of birth, increasing inflammation and detoxifying all at once? First, it's important to recognize that you're entering a different stage of the Protocol. The first stage, Days One through Five, was all about recovery, restoring, and rebuilding your body and energy. The second stage, which encompasses Days Six and Seven, is when the body repeats its seven-day inflammation-detoxification frenzy.

As for what happens on Day Six specifically, you can think of today as the start of the storm. Day Six is when the heavy rains begin, and you start to see flooding—a metaphor that's apt in more ways than one. Let me explain.

On Day Six, your kidneys take over as the star of the show. These little bean-shaped organs kick into high gear today, filtering and flushing out smaller toxins and metabolic waste (substances leftover from cellular processes that the kidneys clear from the blood) in order to prepare for Day Seven—when the liver begins your body's biggest detoxification process. The kidneys undertake some of that detoxification activity today in order to create more room for the liver's massive cleanse tomorrow. In this sense, you can think of the kidneys as the opening act or warm-up band before the big show: They're getting your body ready before the liver has to come on stage and perform all night.

On a normal day, your kidneys filter around two hundred quarts of blood, from which they produce one to two quarts of urine.[1] On Day Six, however, they're filtering much more than that, subsequently producing more urine—why you can expect to have to go to the bathroom more frequently today. The kidneys are filtering and flushing many things that can cause us to retain water, including uric acid and mineral salts like sodium and potassium. This is why

Day Six is like the heavy rains and flooding part of a storm: There are a ton of fluids moving through your body today as the kidneys do their work.

The more metabolic waste, cellular fluid, and smaller toxins that your kidneys filter and flush today, the more toxins your liver will be able to process and purge tomorrow. Every illness, virus, and emotion we ever experience is processed through the liver, which creates a reservoir of toxic debris that can be weeks, months, and even years old. Processing through this waste in the liver is where true healing happens. But if the liver has to spend most of Day Seven filtering smaller toxins and relatively harmless markers like uric acid and mineral salts from cells, it won't have a lot of time to access the stored debris that may be harming your health. That's why it's important to do everything you can today to help support your kidneys.

Your body's inflammation levels are also higher today than they have been all week. This, in combination with the massive filtering and flushing push of the kidneys, can cause many people to feel sluggish, foggy, or groggy today.

Biology: What Happens in Your Body Today

Kidney function peaks on Day Six, as the organs excrete more in quantity and quality than they do all week. They do this by filtering more blood than they normally do, getting rid of excess uric acid, potassium, sodium, and other metabolic waste and mineral salts. Whenever I measure kidney function in my patients on Day Six, their activity is always sky-high, with increased electrolyte excretion.

All this filtering and flushing by your kidneys affects the rest of you in discernible ways. Not only will you likely have to pee more often but you may also feel thirstier, and you're at a much greater risk of dehydration today than any other day of the week. Misbalanced electrolyte levels can also cause headaches and brain fog. Your muscles may also be more sensitive today, as the kidneys pull fluid waste and mineral salts from tissues. This can cause chronic aches and pains to intensify.

Your lymphatic system is busy today, too, collecting and carrying toxins to smaller organs, as well as to the liver. Similarly, liver function continues to intensify, as the body produces more liver enzymes—measurable in blood work—in response to increasing inflammation. About 80 percent of my patients also experience today what I call a "detox belly"—a slight distention of their lower abdomen due to heightened liver function.

Your hormones are also on the rise, including your stress hormone cortisol, along with estrogen and testosterone—all three of which, in excess, can cause inflammation. Other inflammatory markers are also escalating, including interferons—a group of proteins secreted by immune cells to help counter viruses and infection—and C-reactive protein, a protein made by the liver in response to inflammation. Your body's histamine levels also surge today, which can trigger skin sensitivity and increase the likelihood of an adverse reaction to a new food, skin-care product, or other substances in your environment.

Emotions: What Happens in Your Mind Today

The word I hear most often when my patients describe how they feel on Day Six is *hungover*. The description is appropriate: With all the filtering and flushing going on by your kidneys today, in addition to elevated hormone and inflammation levels, you can feel a little worn out, headachy, sluggish, foggy, irritable, overly sensitive, and/or slow, just like you would after a big night out.

Many of my patients also tell me they often feel frustrated today, as though they can't get out of their own way—a sign that you're aware that your body is trying to do something internally, which is cleanse itself. If you're a woman, it's similar to PMS, when you feel tired, irritable, or easily frustrated before getting your period.

Daily Mantra: What to Tell Yourself to Stay Centered and Help Heal

To drive home today's purpose, recognize that as you discard the weight of emotions and conditions that no longer serve you, you're inviting new experiences and opportunities for wellness. Repeat the following mantra when you wake up and whenever you feel uncentered or uncertain throughout the day:

**When I release what no longer serves me,
I give space for new things in life.**

Actions: Best Things to Do Today

1. **Hydrate, hydrate, hydrate.** One of the best ways to support your kidneys today is by drinking more water. Staying hydrated will help the kidneys operate optimally, flushing more metabolic waste and other toxins through urine without having to worry about keeping enough cellular fluid for basic physiological function. If you can, prioritize drinking alkalinized water, which has a slightly higher pH and will prevent acid buildup in your blood. I also recommend drinking water with added electrolytes (but without added sugar) to help balance your electrolytes. Vitaminwater Zero, Smartwater, and even Pedialyte (which has a minimal amount of sugar) are all good choices.

2. **Avoid alcohol and caffeine.** I haven't talked much about the role of alcohol on the Protocol because a few glasses of wine or a cocktail (without any added juices, syrups, or liqueurs) every now and then is fine–as long as you keep it to every now and then (just avoid beer, which contains gluten). But the one day you'll want to restrict all alcohol is Day Six. Not only will booze force your kidneys to work harder but alcohol also dehydrates, creating imbalances in cellular fluid and electrolyte levels. For the same reasons, try to avoid drinking all kinds of caffeine. If you absolutely must have a cup of coffee and don't have any existing kidney problems, limit your intake to no more than one cup today.

3. **Steer clear of stressful situations.** Elevating your blood pressure today will only impair the ability of your kidneys to effectively filter blood. This means you should try to avoid emotionally charged situations or people whenever possible–today is not the day to fire an employee, confront your spouse, tackle financial debt, read a critical email, or have a relationship-defining talk. Stressful situations will also boost your cortisol levels, which are already elevated on Day Six, adding even more inflammation.

HEALTH: MEDICAL TESTS, TREATMENTS, AND THERAPIES TO PRIORITIZE TODAY

1. **Avoid invasive procedures.** While it's okay (but not ideal) to have some kinds of diagnostic tests or small procedures today–think a Pap smear or mole removal–you should avoid major or invasive treatments if you can. More inflammation and the tendency toward dehydration can complicate traumatic interventions like surgery. What's more, most blood work done today may not produce entirely accurate results, due to an increase in metabolic waste and other toxins in your bloodstream.

2. **Get tested for a blood disorder.** While most types of lab work are not advisable today, if you or your doctor suspect you may have a blood disorder, such as a clotting problem or any form of anemia, ask to have your blood drawn on Day Six. Since the kidneys are filtering blood at a greater rate, there's a higher chance that blood work will pick up any problems with your blood cells, platelets, vessels, bone marrow, or the proteins involved in bleeding and clotting.

3. **Schedule genetic work.** This surprises my patients: While most forms of health care aren't advisable on Days Six and Seven, it's actually a great time to have any type of genetic testing done. That's because you have a higher chance of displaying genetic expressions, variants, or anomalies today and tomorrow, when your body is reverting back to the time of your birth and is much more reactive. This increases the chance that DNA and RNA markers will be triggered and expressed.

SELF-CARE: BEST WAYS TO NOURISH YOUR BODY, MIND, AND SPIRIT TODAY

1. **Try a float tank.** Sensory deprivation tank therapy, more commonly known as float tank therapy, has become more popular in recent years as more and more people have realized

all the benefits–physical, mental, and spiritual–of floating weightless in a dark, soundproof tank. That's what happens when you experience the therapy, which uses Epsom salt to help people float in shallow water without any support. The treatment mimics what it's like to be in the womb, helping sync your body with your circaseptan rhythms and prepare to repeat the trauma of birth. More directly, studies show that soaking in Epsom salt can help regulate electrolyte and fluid imbalances, lower blood pressure, ease headaches and muscle pains, and, most important, pull toxins and heavy metals from the blood.[2]

2. **Make your own Epsom salt bath.** Don't have the time, money, or resources for a float tank? No problem. Re-create the experience at home by drawing a warm bath with two cups of Epsom salt. Turn down the lights and close the door before you climb into the tub and soak for at least fifteen minutes. For an added bonus, combine five to twenty drops of lavender essential oil with a small amount of castile oil, all-natural shower gel, or coconut oil and add to the running water. Studies show this essential oil can help reduce aches and pains, mitigate headaches, and soothe frazzled nerves,[3] all of which are common side effects of Day Six. Just be sure to mix your essential oil with a carrier oil or non-water-soluble liquid to prevent concentrated essential oils from sticking to skin, which can cause irritation.

3. **Meditate.** Every day of the week is a good day to meditate on the Protocol. But if you're feeling frustrated today–common for many of my patients–taking ten to twenty minutes to sit quietly with your eyes closed and focus on your breath can help ground you and ease irritation and dissatisfaction.

EXERCISE: BEST WAYS TO MOVE YOUR BODY TODAY

1. **Avoid strenuous activity.** You don't want to do anything today that will cause you to sweat profusely, since perspiring

increases the likelihood of dehydration—the last thing you want to incur on a day when you're trying to support the kidneys. Avoid strenuous or intense workouts, along with hot yoga and outdoor exercise in hot or humid weather. You'll also want to steer clear of activities that might raise your blood pressure, which will also reduce your kidneys' ability to filter and flush toxins.

2. **Do water aerobics.** If you think water aerobics is for the AARP crowd only, you may want to reconsider: The workout can do wonders for your muscle tone, ability to burn fat, and overall cardiovascular function while still being fun, social, and lively, no matter your age. And if you do it on Day Six, you'll reap even more benefits, since you'll still get in a workout that has a low chance of elevated blood pressure and no risk of perspiration. Best of all, it's cathartic to be in any kind of aquatic environment today that mirrors the feeling of being inside the womb.

3. **Try tai chi.** Like water aerobics, tai chi is sweat-free and won't raise your blood pressure. On the contrary, this form of Chinese martial arts is a moving meditation, which will lower your blood pressure while helping you release frustration, eliminate emotional and energetic blockages, and feel more grounded.

Steve's Story: The Power of Day Six

Steve stands out in my roster of patients because, when I first met the thirty-six-year-old, he was unlike almost anyone I'd ever worked with. A young finance professional and bachelor, Steve was primarily interested only in health as a vehicle to help him lift more weights and build muscle mass. He worked out in the gym every single day, which he complemented with a diet of steak, protein shakes, and energy drinks. Despite all this, he was relatively healthy for most of his years—until one day he wasn't.

Steve came to see me after getting sick with one kidney stone after another, some of which were so severe he ended up in the hospital for treatment. At the same time, he also developed gout, a type of inflammatory arthritis that occurs because of too much uric acid in the blood, often caused by poor kidney function and/or a diet rich in red meat. Steve didn't know what was causing his health problems, and his doctors didn't explain—they simply tried to get rid of his symptoms without treating the cause. Although he was taking a fistful of drugs for gout, Steve's symptoms weren't going away, and he routinely experienced swelling in his joints and pressure whenever he had to pee.

When I told Steve about the Protocol, he was skeptical. He'd never been exposed to naturopathic, functional, or integrative medicine and thought the idea of aligning your body with a natural seven-day cycle was woo-woo. But he was willing to try it since nothing else was working—and one of his friends, a professional athlete whom I had also treated, told him that getting on the Protocol helped him perform at an even higher level. To Steve, this meant that even if syncing with his seven-day cycle didn't cure his stones or gout, it could maybe at least help him lift better.

But adopting the Protocol at surface level wasn't going to be enough to stop Steve's stones and gout. I knew that I had to make sure that he did everything right on Day Six, when the kidneys have the greatest opportunity to flush all the salts and uric acid that were causing his stones and gout. This meant absolutely no strenuous weight workouts on Day Six, along with no kinds of caffeine. I also mandated that Steve drink more water every day of the week, paying special attention to his intake on Day Six.

I also made some big changes to Steve's diet, none of which he was particularly happy about at first. I told him he had to reduce his red-meat consumption significantly, swapping out his steaks and burgers for seafood, eggs, and plant-based protein like soy, nuts, and beans. I also told him to say goodbye to his beloved energy drinks, which, with their double whammy of caffeine and sugar, were only dehydrating him further while shocking his adrenal glands—responsible for mitigating the body's stress reaction.

These lifestyle changes weren't easy for Steve, especially giving up the gym on Day Six—he was like an addict scratching at the door to get his fix. He worried he'd lose muscle mass eating only salmon and eggs for protein, and he dreaded Day Six because he knew he couldn't have any coffee.

But in two weeks' time, when his swelling and urination pressure went way for the first time in years, his complaints about the Protocol suddenly subsided. In a few more weeks, Steve had gone more than a month with experiencing a stone—a recent record for him—and he was actually able to lift more in the weight room than he ever had before. That propelled him to continue to follow the Protocol for six months, until his gout completely subsided. At that point, I allowed Steve to start having one cup of coffee on Day Six—by this time, he knew what he had to do to live by the Protocol, and I knew this small addition wouldn't derail his kidney function.

In three years, Steve hasn't had one kidney stone, and his gout hasn't returned. While he doesn't live by the Protocol each and every week, whenever he's off, he says that he's still careful about what he does on Day Six, making sure that he does everything he can to support his kidney function. He also knows that he can fall back on the Protocol whenever he starts to feel unwell or his performance in the weight room declines.

Supplements: Best Nutrients to Take to Support Your Body and Mind Today

On Days Six and Seven, the supplement regimen changes. No matter which health conditions you may be experiencing, you should stop taking *all* supplements recommended for Days One through Five. Instead, take the following three *only*, according to package instructions. These supplements are critical to help the kidneys and liver eliminate as many toxins as possible. For a reminder of why these three supplements are imperative, see page 63.

When you take the following supplements, visualize each one feeding your body's beautiful bud, helping its lush, colorful petals begin to unfurl.

- Milk thistle
- Dandelion root
- Activated charcoal

Diet: Best Foods to Prioritize Today

On Day Six, you'll want to prioritize consuming foods that will help support your kidneys in a major way. The following eight foods include nutrients that will boost kidney function, helping them filter and flush more toxins. They're also all low in phosphorous, a mineral that, in excess, can damage the kidneys. While lean, healthy protein from fish and good fats like the kind found in macadamia nuts are okay in moderation, you'll want to limit how much overall protein and fat you consume today, since both can tax the liver, slowing down your body's ability to detoxify. As a reminder, be sure to avoid all forms of caffeine and alcohol today.

- Cauliflower
- Sea bass
- Garlic
- Cabbage
- Macadamia nuts
- Radishes
- Turnips
- Pineapple

DAY SEVEN: REBIRTH

Day Seven is a big day. It's the biggest day of the entire Protocol. Think of it as the height of the storm, the crescendo in a music piece, the big show, or the marathon you've been training for all week. Today is when your body repeats the trauma of your birth.

As a quick reminder, we repeat the trauma of birth every week because all organisms, including human beings, replicate the actions that help them survive—and the single day when your survival was most in jeopardy was the day on which you were born. It was your make-or-break moment, and the inflammation and detoxification that Little Newborn You initiated were exactly how you were able to make it. By repeating this inflammation-detoxification frenzy and reaping the consequential healing effect, your body ensures its continued survival. The transformation is fast and furious, as your body surges in inflammation and detoxifies in a matter of hours before recovering and beginning the whole seven-day cycle again on Day One.

On Day Seven, every single endogenous chemical peaks in your body—*endogenous* meaning those that the body produces internally, including hormones, immune proteins, cellular waste products, and other possible toxins. This creates a massive amount of inflammation that triggers the liver to go into full detoxification mode to try to lower this inflammation. If it can, the liver will start to process and purge any *exogenous* toxins—those that are produced outside the body that we ingest, breathe, or absorb from food, personal-care products, prescription drugs, and the environment.

Chemicals aren't the only things the liver is working to eradicate today. During its detoxification frenzy, the organ can also break down and eliminate harmful emotions. In addition to physical toxins like ammonia, the liver stores the body's suppressed and sublimated emotions. These feelings have a toxic value, increasing the body's overall inflammatory load. Research from the 1980s by biochemists at St. Paul–Ramsey Medical Center (now known as Regions Hospital) in St. Paul, Minnesota, found that the tears we cry when we're upset contain stress hormones, while reflex tears, or those we produce when our eyes are irritated by an external stimulus, do not.[1] Your liver wants to get rid of harmful emotions, and whatever you can do to support the process will help it get rid of bad feelings and past traumas that, if left in the body too long, can lead to illness and disease.

A great way to help your liver is to live by the Protocol for the six days prior. If your liver and all your other organs and bodily systems are allowed to recover, resettle, restore, rebuild, prepare, and flush, your overall inflammation levels will be lower, and your liver will be primed to kick into full gear on Day Seven to do a really thorough detox. This will allow you to eliminate as many toxins as possible.

Biology: What Happens in Your Body Today

On Day Seven, all the endogenous chemicals that have been slowly rising inside you since the night of Day Five—including histamine; the hormones cortisol, estrogen, testosterone, and adrenaline; cellular waste products like ammonia; and proteins like interferons—suddenly spike. At the same time, your body's viral load surges, as some of the 380 trillion viruses living inside you at any given time become more active. This causes a massive increase in inflammation, which drives up blood pressure.

Your body eliminated some inflammation on Day Six, when the kidneys filtered and flushed smaller toxins and metabolic waste. On Day Seven, the liver now takes over to carry out the Cleanse, breaking down and getting rid of the endogenous chemicals that cause a weekly inflammation surge. After the liver processes them, these endogenous toxins go to the kidneys to be eliminated as urine or through the intestinal tract to be excreted as stool.

During detoxification, your liver will also try to get rid of as many exogenous toxins as it can, including thousands of foreign chemicals circulating in the body at any given time, such as those we consume through foods like refined sugar, gluten, dairy proteins (casein and whey), and alcohol, all of which have an inflammatory effect. It also includes lab-engineered chemicals found in the foods we eat, like artificial dyes, emulsifiers, pesticides, and hormones, along with toxins found in personal-care products like creams, lotions, and makeup—all of which add up to a significant amount, as the average woman rubs more than five hundred synthetic chemicals into her skin every day.[2] We're also exposed to thousands of chemicals in our homes, offices, and the outside world every day, along with any prescription and over-the-counter drugs like ibuprofen or antacids that we take, which break down into toxic byproducts.

While it's nearly impossible to avoid all toxins in food, products, drugs, and the environment, you can help your body get rid of them more quickly, effectively, and easily by doing everything you can to support the liver. One of the best ways to do this is to create less endogenous inflammation in the first place. Avoiding common toxins found in food, like sugar, gluten, and dairy proteins, is also key, as is taking potent anti-inflammatory supplements Days One through Five and the three detoxifying nutrients I recommend on page 69 Days Six and Seven. All these steps can also help prevent or reverse nonalcoholic fatty liver disease (NAFLD), a condition that affects nearly one-third of all Americans.[3] NAFLD, in which the liver stores too much fat due to factors such as obesity, poor diet, and insulin resistance, can eventually cause fatigue, pain, and even liver scarring and failure.

Your liver isn't just busy detoxifying today—it's also rebuilding itself. The liver is the only organ that regenerates: You could have two-thirds of your liver removed, and it would grow back completely in seven days.[4] While no one is removing your liver, it's still programmed to regenerate every seven days by manufacturing healthy new cells from the inside out. This is why I tell my patients the liver is the hardest-working organ and why they need to try to do everything possible to support it, especially on Day Seven.

Outside the liver, your immune system is on full alert today, as it responds to inflammation like it would any illness or infection. This isn't a bad thing: The immune response helps your body heal. Your red and white blood cell counts also climb upward today in order to help your immune system fight off inflammation.

Many people can experience the symptoms of a detox belly today, when bloating increases due to heightened liver activity (this is the same reason we feel bloated after a big night of drinking). Because inflammatory levels are higher throughout the body, including in the brain, it's also normal to feel more brain fog and less mental focus, clarity, and acuity on Day Seven.

Emotions: What Happens in Your Mind Today

Day Seven can be an energy roller coaster, depending on how your body responds to the Cleanse. Many people feel tired, as though they've been hit by a ton of bricks or like they're just getting over a bad cold or the flu. Others, however, feel all gassed up, as the healing process gives them a second wind.

From an emotional perspective, Day Seven can be turbulent. As your liver processes old emotions and traumas, these feelings surface in order to be broken down and discharged. This can trigger many different emotional responses. You may feel like crying or pounding your fists against the wall for no reason, for example, or you may also feel elated. No matter what emotions come up, I encourage you to embrace them and remain nonjudgmental. It's up to you whether you try to unpack them via journaling or meditation of if you simply allow yourself the space to feel and heal.

Daily Mantra: What to Tell Yourself to Stay Centered and Help Heal

To drive home today's purpose, tell yourself that you are worthy of wellness and that all areas of your life can flow more easily from this source of wellness. Repeat the following mantra when you wake up and whenever you feel uncentered or uncertain throughout the day:

All of nature is in perfect order, and I am a part of that order.

Actions: Best Things to Do Today

1. **Journal.** Day Seven opens the floodgates of your emotional past, allowing old traumas and feelings to work their way out of your body. You don't have to analyze what every emotion might mean, but writing down how you feel can help your brain recognize and identify feelings, consequently giving your liver the push it might need to release them. I've also found that journaling helps me make sense of the chaos inside today and increases mental clarity at a time when I often feel scatterbrained.

2. **Listen to your body.** Some people have a lot of energy today; others don't have any at all. No matter which camp you fall

into—and it may change week to week—listen to your body. If you're tired and need more rest, take it. Or if you feel energized and want to tackle your to-do list, by all means, do so. The critical thing is to tune in to what your body is trying to tell you—something so few of us do on a regular basis. Practicing the fine art of listening to your body can better align you with what's happening inside and help your liver work more effectively so you can heal.

3. **Be open to epiphanies.** Energies shift today, as you release stored toxins and suppressed emotions, which can lead to new insight. You may not have a ton of mental clarity today, but you'll likely feel frustrated, which can trigger new revelations about what you like and don't like about your current situation. As the body eliminates toxins and emotions, you may also find your priorities changing, as you realize which external things are worth holding on to and what is better off released.

HEALTH: MEDICAL TESTS, TREATMENTS, AND THERAPIES TO PRIORITIZE TODAY

1. **Avoid invasive procedures.** You'll want to avoid invasive procedures like major surgery today if at all possible. High inflammation levels on Day Seven increase the risk of complications while reducing the chance for success. What's more, invasive procedures can interrupt or distract your body from the detoxification process.

2. **Reschedule blood work and diagnostic testing.** You'll also want to avoid most types of blood work and diagnostic testing today, as elevated inflammation levels can obscure results.

3. **Consider colonics if you've done them before.** While a colonic is certainly an invasive procedure, if you're used to

receiving them, having one today can speed toxin removal. When you get a colonic, otherwise known as colon cleansing therapy, a tube is inserted into your rectum and warm water is pumped into your body to flush the intestines. Typically, people receive colonics to help remove toxins from the body, as well as because they believe it can improve digestion, limit bloating, speed weight loss, and treat some health issues like arthritis and skin conditions.[5] If you've never had one, don't try the procedure for the first time on Day Seven—schedule it for Days Two through Four to see first how your body adapts. On the other hand, if you're a veteran colonic user, you can experiment with the procedure on Day Seven, but definitely pay close attention to how you feel afterward. If the treatment leaves you fatigued or run-down, omit it from your Day Seven regime. Otherwise, if the procedure helps you feel regenerated, colonics might be a great way to support your liver.

SELF-CARE: BEST WAYS TO NOURISH YOUR BODY, MIND, AND SPIRIT TODAY

1. **Do a foot soak.** Soaking your feet in warm water with Epsom salts and essential oils like eucalyptus (mixed beforehand with a carrier oil or liquid bath product) can draw impurities from the feet, where we store many toxins, doing some of the work the liver would otherwise have to do. Epsom salt foot soaks also help the body absorb magnesium, which reduces inflammation, according to studies.[6] I like them on Day Seven because they're also relaxing and require little work, making them more accessible and practical for those feeling low on energy today.

2. **Be as indulgent as you want.** Comfort is king on Day Seven, so I always tell my patients to do whatever they need to in order to make themselves feel as relaxed as possible today. For some, that means drawing a bubble bath and listening to relaxing

music; for others, it might mean sitting on the couch and drinking hot tea. But whatever you want to do, give yourself permission to indulge today.

3. **Continue to hydrate.** While your kidneys aren't filtering and flushing as much through your urine today as they were yesterday, you'll still want to focus on hydration. Optimal hydration increases liver function and helps the body eliminate as much as possible.

EXERCISE: BEST WAYS TO MOVE YOUR BODY TODAY

1. **Don't do any strenuous exercise.** If Day Six isn't great for intense or high-impact workouts, Day Seven is even worse. That's because your body is even more inflamed today, increasing your risk of injury and slowing down recovery time. If you work out too hard or too long, it can also interrupt or distract your body from its detoxification process. If you feel like a million bucks on Day Seven, concentrate on channeling that energy inward to heal your body.

2. **Take a brisk walk.** Just because hard workouts are off the calendar today doesn't mean you have to sit on the couch morning, noon, and night. Going for a brisk walk will increase blood flow to organs, including the liver, helping you get rid of more toxins more quickly. Taking a walk can also clear your mind and rebalance turbulent emotions while giving you the headspace you might need to recognize new insights.

3. **Stretch.** Like walking, stretching also increases blood flow to the liver and other organs, helping the body detoxify. A good stretch session also stimulates the lymphatic system, encouraging lymph to carry toxins more easily out of the body.

Mark's Story: The Power of Day Seven

The Protocol isn't only for adults. Teaching children and young adults to live in harmony with their seven-day cycle can establish healthy cellular patterns while the body is still growing and prevent toxin storage that can lead to disease later in life. I've also found that the Protocol helps kids focus better in and out of school, whether they're in class, playing sports, learning an instrument, or participating in another creative or intellectual pursuit.

I started working with fourteen-year-old Mark after his parents reached out to me because they were worried about his health. Mark was a talented and passionate golfer, but lately his joints would swell whenever he played, his scoring had taken a nosedive, and he would often come back from the course irritable and unable to sleep that night. He was already on the prescription sleep aid Lunesta and had seen an osteopath and other doctors to try to address his joint issues, but nothing was working. When his parents spoke with another member of the country club where Mark played and learned how I had helped her lose weight just by getting on the Protocol, they called to see if I could also help their son with his issues.

The easy part about Mark was that his diet was already ideal, especially for a fourteen-year-old boy. His parents were extremely health conscious, so there was no sugary or processed junk in his house, and family meals were usually seafood or another lean protein with lots of fresh vegetables, and a modicum of healthy, whole grains. Mark's problem, however, wasn't what he was eating but what he was doing—and particularly what he was doing on Day Seven.

As it turned out, Mark's Day Seven was Saturday, which was also the one day he could play golf for as long and as hard as he wanted. While the sport isn't necessarily strenuous, Mark took it to the next level, sometimes playing thirty-six holes in one day before practicing his swing at the range. He was exerting himself more on Day Seven than any other day of the week, which was driving up his inflammation and interfering with his body's ability to detoxify. The result was a swollen right ankle, a swollen left knee, reduced athletic performance, increased irritability, and sleeplessness, as his body struggled to battle inflammation overload.

Since Mark had school during the week and the course was closed to younger patrons on Sunday, Saturday was the only day he could play for as long as he wanted. This made it difficult to convince him to give up the game altogether on Saturdays, but eventually I won him over, persuading him to focus his energy on playing Tuesday and Wednesday instead—his Days Three and Four—when his muscles and joints would have much greater blood flow and lower levels of inflammation.

Within weeks after Mark switched his play schedule, his golf game turned around. The swelling in both his knee and ankle receded while his score shot up. He no longer felt irritable—not just because his golf game had improved but also because he wasn't routinely exacerbating his inflammation levels. His sleep also stabilized, so much so that we weaned him off of the Lunesta. Even the teenage acne he had started to subside. Six months later, he told me getting on the Protocol transformed his game.

Supplements: Best Nutrients to Take to Support Your Body and Mind Today

When you take your supplements, visualize your body's bud bursting open into a flower, thanks to the nutrients you've fed it this week, as it's now ready to display its full magnitude and beauty.

- Milk thistle
- Dandelion root
- Activated charcoal

Diet: Best Foods to Prioritize Today

Your liver is working harder than it has all week, which is why you'll want to try to do what you can to nourish and fuel the organ today. At the same time, you'll also want to prioritize foods that aid in the detoxification process, off-loading some of the liver's work. The following seven foods all boost liver function and detoxification efforts. But today, it's not just about what you eat but what you don't eat, so be careful to minimize foods that impair liver function or slow detoxification, like sugar, gluten, dairy, processed items, alcohol, and caffeine. If you like coffee, however, go ahead and have one cup of black coffee today, which will help speed detoxification—just be sure to keep it to one cup to avoid taxing the liver.

- Grapefruit
- Garlic
- Almonds
- Black coffee
- Green tea
- Dandelion greens
- Beets

MAINTAINING THE PROTOCOL

CHAPTER 14

You've learned a lot about the Protocol over the last thirteen chapters, and I hope you've found it as fascinating as I do. But with so much information specific to each day, how do you actually maintain the Protocol week to week to week? That's what this chapter is all about. I've helped hundreds of patients adopt and follow the Protocol for months, even years, and I have lots of tips and tricks that will make the plan easy to follow, no matter who you are, how healthy you might already be, what you do for a living, or what kind of lifestyle you currently lead.

Why Maintain the Protocol?

The Protocol can change your life in one week's time by helping you align with your body's natural biorhythms, thereby reducing inflammation and triggering a deeper detoxification than you've likely ever experienced before. But maintaining the Protocol for at least one month's time (four seven-day cycles) is when real miracles happen. Here's why. The first week or two after you sync with your circaseptan rhythms, your body reduces and eliminates the natural inflammation that occurs as part of your seven-day cycle. Only after your body gets a handle on its weekly inflammation can it begin to address and lower the underlying, chronic inflammation that causes most health issues, whether you're trying to heal a serious disease like diabetes or a relatively minor ailment like hair loss. As a reminder, the body is always evolving and nothing is permanent—you do have the power and potential to heal yourself, so honor this process and give it the time, effort, and attention it deserves.

Another reason the one-month mark is so powerful is because that's how long it usually takes to break a bad habit or form a healthy new one. This can be key since it's not easy at first to sync your diet with your seven-day cycle— oftentimes, it takes time to learn tricks of the trade and how to substitute healing foods that are just as delicious and convenient for proinflammatory ones that are packed with added sugar, refined carbs, red meat, dairy, and other standard American staples. Similarly, learning to structure your daily routine around your body's needs rather than letting external sources dictate what you do can be challenging, as can remembering to take your supplements when you haven't made them a habit yet. What I tend to see is that people get better at the Protocol the longer they follow it, as parameters of the plan become habit and second nature.

There's also a universal synergy in following your seven-day rhythms for one month. When you do so, you're no different than the moon and tide. You give yourself the same duration to heal as the natural rotation of a woman's fertility cycle or a man's rise and fall in testosterone.

The longer you follow the Protocol, the more benefits you'll see, too. But I want to remind you of something I said in chapter 6: Focus on progress over perfection. Instead of starting with the intent to maintain the Protocol forever and ever, make it your goal to do so for four weeks. And at that point, set another two-, four-, or six-week goal.

How to Maintain the Protocol

Nothing about your body or your health is permanent—you have the power and potential right now to change what you want about your physical and emotional well-being. At the same time, your current state of health and being didn't happen overnight, and you're not necessarily going to transform them overnight, either. Miracles can take time, but time isn't synonymous with laborious or impossible. You can do this and live your life according to the Protocol for more than one week. Here's how.

Simplify the steps. The easiest way to adopt and sustain the Protocol is to simplify it, especially as you learn the ins and outs of the plan. Here, I've broken the plan down into its three main components, or what I like to call the three *d*'s: daily habits, diet, and dietary supplements. These are the components to focus on every day and week as you follow the Protocol.

Daily habits are the activities you do, personal interactions you have, and lifestyle choices and medical decisions you make on a regular basis. This includes how you exercise, the way you interact with other people, the tasks and chores you decide to tackle in the office or at home, the physical and mental stress you expose yourself to, and the medical therapies and treatments you opt to receive.

When you follow the Protocol, you'll want to modify as many of your daily habits as you can to sync with your seven-day cycle so that what you do comple-ments what's happening inside your body on that day of the week. To help you do this, I recommend rereading each day's chapter the night before during the first two weeks you begin the plan. Afterward, you'll likely develop a routine and a better understanding of the Protocol so that you won't need to remind yourself how to tailor your activities to each specific day.

The Protocol should also become second nature over time. Your body is pro-grammed to want to align with your natural circaseptan rhythms just like it's designed to get up in the morning with the sun and go to bed at night, according to our internal circadian clocks.

During your first few weeks on the plan, however, you may find it helpful to remind yourself of the primary theme of each day. For example, the theme of Day One is recovery, so no matter what you do that day, prioritize supporting physi-cal and mental recovery—or at the very least, try to avoid activities, interactions, or interventions that will inhibit recovery. The theme of Day Two, on the other hand, is resettle, meaning your body has gone back to baseline, and you'll have more energy and physical bandwidth to travel, tackle projects, take on stressful conversations, make big decisions, and work out strenuously.

Here's a reminder of the theme of all seven days:

- Day One: recover
- Day Two: resettle
- Day Three: restore
- Day Four: rebuild
- Day Five: prepare
- Day Six: flush
- Day Seven: rebirth

Think of Days Two through Five as your high-energy, high-impact days, when most forms of exercise, medical treatments, interpersonal interactions, and other types of potentially stressful activities (whether positive or negative) won't overwhelm your body's seven-day inflammation cycle. Days Six, Seven, and One, however, are when it's critical to keep things light and easy, avoiding most kinds of physical and mental stress, including travel, strenuous activity, invasive medical procedures, tense conversations, or risky decisions.

Diet is critical on the Protocol. As you've read, what you eat can drastically reduce your body's inflammatory load. When you consume certain foods at spe-cific times, you help boost the body's seven-day inflammation response while giving your cells the nutrition they need on the days they need it the most. But what you don't eat is just as important, since so many of the foods commonly found in the standard American diet drive up inflammation levels significantly and interfere with your body's detoxification process. Foods to minimize on the Protocol include processed items with added sugar or refined carbs, red meat, cow's dairy, nightshade vegetables, and corn (see pages 60–63 for why you should minimize these foods).

The Protocol is not an elimination diet, meaning you don't eliminate these foods for seven days, then reintroduce them. Added sugar, refined carbs, red meat, cow's dairy, nightshade veggies, and corn are problematic for all people, no matter who you are or what other food sensitivities you might have, because they can and will drive up inflammation in everyone. That means you should continue to minimize these proinflammatory foods as much as possible as you continue to follow the Protocol. At the same time, I understand these foods make up the majority of our diet and avoiding them altogether can be tricky, if not impossible. That's why I use the word *minimize* instead of *avoid*: As long as you minimize proinflammatory foods most of the time, you can still celebrate with a piece of birthday cake or have a cheeseburger at your friend's barbecue—it won't undo everything you've worked toward. Aim to follow the eighty-twenty rule: Prioritize healing foods 80 percent of the time and indulge in proinflammatory foods no more than 20 percent of the time. For more tips on how to maintain the eating plan on the Protocol, see pages 55–56.

Dietary supplements aren't absolutely necessary on the Protocol, but I highly recommend taking them as outlined in chapter 4. (If you choose not to take supplements, the aforementioned dietary changes are even more important.) The supplements suggested Days One through Five are potent anti-inflammatories that will lower and reset the body's inflammatory load. This means your kidneys and liver will have less to process and eliminate on Days Six and Seven as part of your natural inflammation cycle, allowing them to tackle preexisting toxins and other inflammatory markers caused by or exacerbating any illness, ailment, or disease you might have.

The supplements recommended for Days Six and Seven play a different role. During the Cleanse, your kidneys and liver are busy breaking down and excreting excess chemicals and metabolic waste created over your seven-day cycle, along with any older toxins they have the bandwidth to access. Supplementing with milk thistle, dandelion root, and activated charcoal—three of the strongest natural detoxicants—can support these organs and help the body eliminate even more toxins.

Remind yourself why you want to do this. Are you suffering from a chronic ailment, illness, or disease that won't go away no matter what you do or which treatments you try? Are you uncomfortable about how you look or feel in your own body? Do you wish you had more energy or just weren't so tried all the time? Are you struggling with depression, anxiety, or mental clarity? Are you concerned about a family history of cancer, heart disease, diabetes, or dementia? Reminding yourself on a daily basis why you adopted the Protocol in the first place can help you stay focused and committed.

Remember, too, that the Protocol gives you an incredible opportunity every day to get a little bit healthier. Each day, you have the chance to support your body. No big, sweeping, or overwhelming changes are necessary—instead, you simply make a daily commitment to do what you can to nurture your body's specific functions on that particular day. I've learned that small, daily changes are how progress happens, and having a specific, reasonable time period in which to accomplish your goals can make your journey to better health and wellness easier and more sustainable.

Record and celebrate your progress. You know that when you see the same person every day, it can be difficult to recognize subtle changes like a hair trimming or a five-pound weight gain or loss. The same is true of ourselves. Since we see and live in our own bodies every day, it can be hard to realize if and when we start to look or feel better. That's why I recommend journaling how you feel *before* you start the Protocol, then doing so on Day Five every week thereafter, noting any improvements in sleep, digestion, energy, mental outlook, stress levels, weight, appearance, or symptoms associated with an ailment, illness, or disease. Reread your initial entry every week and take the time to recognize the progress you've made. Celebrate these improvements and use them as motivation to keep going.

Don't restrict. The Protocol isn't a diet—it's a lifestyle plan that uses daily habits, food, and dietary supplements to align you with your seven-day cycle. That's why I use the terms *prioritize* and *minimize* when it comes to which foods to consume rather than the words *only eat* or *avoid*. If you have some candy, pizza, or a cinnamon roll every now and then, you won't undo or entirely derail your progress. I even recommended the best time of the week to enjoy proinflammatory foods, which is Day Five, or right before your body begins to detoxify, which will give it a chance to clear the inflammation from whatever you eat.

What I don't want you to do, however, is to perceive any food as off-limits. As soon as you do, you'll be more tempted to consume it, overeat, or give up on healthy eating altogether, studies show.[1] Instead of restricting or eliminating certain foods, accept that you're an adult who can eat whatever you want while prioritizing the foods you know will heal your body, like green vegetables, seafood, citrus and other fruits, beans, nuts, whole grains, honey, dark chocolate, and even coffee. For more tips and tricks on following an anti-inflammatory diet, see the text on personalizing the Protocol for weight loss on page 53.

Treat supplements like insurance. Some people stop taking supplements after they start to see results on the Protocol because they assume they don't need them anymore. Others stop taking them after just a few days because they believe supplements should work like prescription medications, with immediate results. Neither is a good approach. Think of supplements like health insurance or paying to put high-octane fuel into a high-performance car: Doing so is a relatively easy, low-effort way to safeguard and supercharge your health and physical and mental performance. If you suddenly stop having health insurance or using high-octane fuel, your safety net or chance for optimal performance drops out from under you, even if you're already healthy. The same is true of supplements.

I also want to underscore that supplements aren't pharmaceutical drugs—a good thing, since most supplements don't have as many harmful side effects or the potential toxicity that most prescription drugs do. But because supplements aren't designed to wallop your body or suppress your symptoms, most don't work instantaneously—they take time to build up in the body. And everyone's bodies are different when it comes to how we process nutrients. Before you decide whether a supplement is ineffective for you, take it regularly for at least three months if you don't have an underlying illness and at least six months if you're dealing with a chronic disease.

Focus on two of the three *d*'s (daily habits, diet, and dietary supplements) on the days when it's impossible to nail all three. I totally get that some days will be more hectic than others, and you can't upend your work schedule, avoid traveling, or cancel a stressful meeting just because the Protocol suggests doing so. On those days when your daily habits aren't modifiable, double down on eating right and taking your supplements. Similarly, if you fall off the food wagon and end up eating lots of proinflammatory items, make sure you're doing everything possible to align your daily habits and supplement regimen with what's happening in your body that day.

Break it down. If you're struggling to maintain the Protocol, break it down into the smallest denominator, or the component that's posing the biggest problems for you. For example, is your work schedule the biggest roadblock to your ability to maintain your seven-day cycle? If so, which part of your job is the least modifiable to the Protocol? Or are you constantly tempted by proinflammatory foods? If so, which items in particular? When you repackage the problem into a smaller box, you'll likely discover solutions to address the issue. For example, if you feel deprived because you're not eating cheese and it's causing you to over-indulge in or overeat other proinflammatory foods, try having a small piece of cheese every day to see if that solves the problem.

Be patient. Whenever you adopt a new routine or diet, you have to give it time to work, and the Protocol is no different. After one week on the plan, you can expect to feel increased mental clarity, improved digestion, a greater sense of accomplishment, and a better connection with your body and yourself—these effects will increase and multiply the longer you stay on the plan. Of course, like everything else in life, there can be bumps along the way—if and when you do face a setback, look at it as an opportunity to reinvest in your health.

Prioritize your health. The greatest things in life often require sacrifices. To optimize your health and well-being, you may need to minimize or forgo other activities. That's okay. As the saying goes, great achievement always requires great sacrifices.

ACKNOWLEDGMENTS

As with all things in life, this work is a bittersweet culmination of my mind, body, and spirit. I know within every fragment of my being a few things: The human body can correct anything with the permission of the soul; our bodies have and always will support us to whatever extent we allow them to thrive; there is far more that remains unknown about the body than we currently understand; and everyone has the ability to heal themselves.

I want to extend my heartfelt gratitude to everyone who has always been and will be part of my soul tribe—you know who you are.

Eternal thanks to the team at Simon & Schuster, to the incredible Leah Miller for your vision, and to Nena Madonia Oshman and everyone at Dupree Miller & Associates for your enduring support. And a heartfelt thanks to my writer, Sarah Toland.

I have total admiration for the three most important humans in my world: Tucker, Mia, and Sullivan. It's not easy having a crazy, mad-scientist, hippie mom. You guys handle it well.

I also want to thank my angel godmother, Margaret, who first taught me the power of self-healing through nature and named each of her flower bushes after the children she loved. I now have a peony bush named Margaret.

To my teacher Wayne Dyer: I feel you every day.

And finally, to those of you reading this now whom I haven't met but someday will, with any luck: This is the beginning of the most important, intimate conversation you will ever have with your body. Ask for what you need from it and listen carefully for the answers. Your body has been waiting your entire lifetime to help you heal.

NOTES

Introduction

1. Simon Worrall, "How 40,000 Tons of Cosmic Dust Falling to the Earth Affects You and Me," *National Geographic*, January 28, 2015, https://www.nationalgeographic.com/news/2015/01/150128-big-bang-universe-supernova-astrophysics-health-space-ngbooktalk/.

2. Josh Hrala, "Scientists Have Found a Bizarre Similarity Between Human Cells and Neutron Stars," *Science Alert*, November 3, 2016, https://www.sciencealert.com/scientists-have-found-a-structural-similarity-between-human-cells-and-neutron-stars.

Chapter 1: The Science of Sevens

1. Fangyi Gu et al., "Total and Cause-Specific Mortality of U.S. Nurses Working Rotating Night Shifts," *American Journal of Preventative Medicine* 58, no. 3 (March 2015): 241–52, https://doi.org/10.1016/j.amepre.2014.10.018.

2. Phillipa J. Karoly et al., "Circadian and Circaseptan Rhythms in Human Epilepsy: A Respective Cohort Study," *Lancet Neurology* 17, no. 11 (November 2018): 977–985, https://doi.org/10.1016/S1474-4422(18)30274-6.

3. John W. Ayers et al., "What's the Healthiest Day?: Circaseptan (Weekly) Rhythms in Healthy Consideration," *American Journal of Preventative Medicine* 47, no. 1 (July 2014): 73–76, DOI: 10.1016/j.amepre.2014.02.003.

4. "Time-Sensitive Clues about Cardiovascular Risk," *Harvard Heart Letter*, Harvard Health Publishing, Harvard Medical School, https://www.health.harvard.edu/heart-health/time-sensitive-clues-about-cardiovascular-risk.

5. Karoly et al., "Circadian and Circaseptan Rhythms," 977–85.

6. Francis Levi and Franz Halberg, "Circaseptan (About-7-Day) Bioperiodicity—Spontaneous and Reactive—and the Search for Pacemakers," *Ricerca in clinica e in laboratorio* 12 (April 1982): 323, https://link.springer.com/article/10.1007/BF02909422.

7. David Adam, "Core Concept: Emerging Science of Chronotherapy Offers Big Opportunities to Optimize Drug Delivery," *Proceedings of the National Academy of Sciences of the United States of America* 116, no. 44 (October 2019): 21957–21959, DOI: 10.1073/pnas.1916118116.

8. David Montaigne et al., "Daytime Variation of Perioperative Myocardial Injury in Cardiac Surgery and Its Prevention by Rev-Erb Antagonism: A Single-Center Propensity-Matched Cohort Study and a Randomized Study," *Lancet* 391, no. 10115 (January 2018): 59–69, https://doi.org/10.1016/S0140-6736(17)32132-3.

9. Adam, "Core Concept," 21957–59.

10. Lynne Peeples, "Medicine's Secret Ingredient—It's in the Timing," *Nature* 556, no. 7701 (April 2018): 290–292, DOI: 10.1038/d41586-018-04600-8.

11. Richard Gray, "Take Aspirin before Bed to Cut Morning Heart Attack Risk," *Telegraph*, November 19, 2013, https://www.telegraph.co.uk/news/health/news/10461007/Take-aspirin-before-bed-to-cut-morning-heart-risk.html.

12. David Leaf, "Class Act: Do Statins Always Have to Be Taken in the Evening?" *Clinical Correlations*, January 10, 2008, https://www.clinicalcorrelations.org/2008/01/10/class-act-morning-versus-evening-administration-of-statins/.

13. Eve Simmons and Roger Dobson, "Never Take Blood Pressure Pills in the Morning and Never Pop Paracetamol before Lunch . . . So When IS the Right Time to Take Your Tablets?" *Daily Mail*, September 21, 2019, https://www.dailymail.co.uk/health/article-7489191/Why-paracetamol-never-taken-lunchtime.html.

14. Ibid.

15. The Nobel Prize in Physiology or Medicine in 2017, "Discoveries of Molecular Mechanisms Controlling the Circadian Rhythm," accessed May 4, 2021, https://www.nobelprize.org/prizes/medicine/2017/advanced-information/.

16. Konstantin Bikos, "Why Does a Week Have Seven Days?" timeanddate.com, accessed May 4, 2021, https://www.timeanddate.com/calendar/days/7-days-week.html.

17. Linda Geddes, "The Mind-Altering Power of the Moon," *BBC Future*, July 31, 2019, https://www.bbc.com/future/article/20190731-is-the-moon-impacting-your-mood-and-wellbeing.

18. I. Stewart, "Number Symbolism," *Encyclopedia Britannica*, November 4, 2020, https://www.britannica.com/topic/number-symbolism/7.

19. Javier Barbuzano, "Understanding How the Intestine Replaces and Repairs Itself, *Harvard Gazette*, July 14, 2017, https://news.harvard.edu/gazette/story/2017/07/understanding-how-the-intestine-replaces-and-repairs-itself/.

20. "Conception: How It Works," University of California San Francisco Health, accessed April 7, 2021, https://www.ucsfhealth.org/education/conception-how-it-works.

21. "Prenatal Form and Function—The Making of an Earth Suit," The Endowment for Human Development, accessed April 7, 2021, https://www.ehd.org/dev_article_unit1.php#implantationbegin.

22. "Female Hormone Cycle," Hormonology, accessed April 7, 2021, https://www.myhormonology.com/learn/female-hormone-cycle/.

23. Ibid.

24. Ibid.

25. Ibid.

26. Erhard Haus, "Chronobiology of the Immune System," in *Military Strategies for Sustainment of Nutrition and Immune Function in the Field*, Institute of Medicine (Washington DC: National Academies Press, 1999), https://www.ncbi.nlm.nih.gov/books/NBK230982/.

27. Ibid.

28. Brendon J. Coventry et al., "CRP Identifies Homeostatic Immune Oscillations in Cancer Patients: A Potential Treatment Targeting Tool?" *Journal of Translational Medicine* 7, no. 102 (November 2009), DOI:10.1186/1479-5876-7-102.

29. Ibid.

30. "Immune Cycle," Grace Gawler Institute, accessed April 7, 2021, https://www
    .gracegawlerinstitute.com/immune-cycle-registry/.
31. Haus, "Chronobiology of the Immune System."
32. Cher Enderby and Cesar Kelly, "An Overview of Immunosuppression in Solid
    Organ Transplantation," *American Journal of Managed Care* 21, no. 1 (January
    2015): S12–S23, https://www.ajmc.com/view/ace022_jan15_enderby.
33. Erika McCormick, "Hidden Rhythms of Life: Understanding Circaseptan
    Rhythms and Their Commonality in Diverse Life Forms," *Rhodes Journal of
    Biological Science* 32 (Spring 2017): 28–35.
34. "Circadian and Circaseptan Rhythms in Human Epilepsy," EpilepsyU, September 13,
    2018, https://epilepsyu.com/circadian-and-circaseptan-rhythms-in-human-epilepsy/.
35. Ibid.
36. Ibid.
37. "The '7 Day COVID-19 Crash,'" *Short Wave*, NPR, April 10, 2020, https://www
    .npr.org/2020/04/09/831257636/the-7-day-covid-19-crash.
38. Ming Jiang et al., "A Research on the Relationship between Ejaculation and Serum
    Testosterone Level in Men," *Journal of Zhejiang University Science* 4, no. 2 (March/
    April 2003): 236–40, DOI: 10.1631/jzus.2003.0236.
39. Guy Winch, "Seven Reasons We Are Captivated by the Number Seven," *Psychology
    Today*, June 27, 2015, https://www.psychologytoday.com/us/blog/the-squeaky
    -wheel/201506/seven-reasons-we-are-captivated-the-number-seven.
40. Ibid.
41. "The Magical Qualities of the Number 7," Diversions, NPR, July 7, 2007, https://
    www.npr.org/templates/story/story.php?storyId=11803762.
42. Michele Migliore, Gaspare Novara, and Domenico Tegolo, "Single Neuron
    Binding Properties and the Magical Number 7," *Hippocampus* 18, no. 11 (2008):
    1122–30, DOI: 10.1002/hipo.20480.
43. Business Wire, "FranklinCovey and Simon & Schuster Release New Edition of
    Stephen Covey's *The 7 Habits of Highly Effective People*, with Personal Insights
    from Son, Sean Covey," May 19, 2020, https://www.businesswire.com/news
    /home/20200519005425/en/FranklinCovey-and-Simon-Schuster-Release-New
    -Edition-of-Stephen-Covey%E2%80%99s-The-7-Habits-of-Highly-Effective
    -People-With-Personal-Insights-from-Son-Sean-Covey.
44. Alex Bellos, "'Seven' Triumphs in Poll to Discover World's Favourite Number,"
    Guardian, April 8, 2014, https://www.theguardian.com/science/alexs-adventures
    -in-numberland/2014/apr/08/seven-worlds-favourite-number-online-survey.
45. Ibid.
46. "Understanding Our Bodies' 7 Year Cycles," Angea, March 20, 2017, http://angea
    .com.au/7-year-cycles/.
47. "Explaining the Ayurvedic Prakriti or Body Constitutions or Body Types!"
    Ayusante, accessed April 7, 2021, http://www.ayusante.com/articles/21.
48. F. Galis, "Why Do Almost All Mammals Have Seven Cervical Vertebrae?
    Developmental Constraints, Hox Genes, and Cancer," *Journal of Experimental
    Zoology* 285, no. 1 (April 1999): 19–26, https://pubmed.ncbi.nlm.nih
    .gov/10327647/.

Chapter 2: Understanding Your Seven-Day Cycle

1. "Health Concerns About Dairy," Physicians Committee for Responsible Medicine, accessed April 7, 2021, https://www.pcrm.org/good-nutrition/nutrition -information/health-concerns-about-dairy.
2. "Meat, Fish & Dairy," World Cancer Research Fund, accessed April 7, 2021, https://www.wcrf.org/dietandcancer/exposures/meat-fish-dairy.
3. "Chronic Illness and Mental Health: Recognizing and Treating Depression," National Institute of Mental Health, accessed April 7, 2021, https://www .nimh.nih.gov/health/publications/chronic-illness-mental-health/index .shtml#:~:text=People%20with%20depression%20have%20an,for%20 osteoporosis%20relative%20to%20others.
4. "Past Trauma May Haunt Your Health," *Harvard Women's Health Watch*, February 2019, https://www.health.harvard.edu/diseases-and-conditions/past-trauma -may-haunt-your-future-health#:~:text=Medical%20conditions%20resulting%20 from%20trauma&text=Early%20childhood%20trauma%20is%20a,stroke%2C%20 cancer%2C%20and%20obesity.
5. Lauri Nummenmaa et al., "Bodily Maps of Emotions," *Proceedings of the National Academy of Sciences of the United States of America* 111, no. 2 (November 2013): 646–51, https://doi.org/10.1073/pnas.1321664111.
6. Stephanie Eckelkamp, "Can Trauma Really Be 'Stored' in the Body?" Mindbodygreen, October 9, 2019, https://www.mindbodygreen.com/articles/can -trauma-be-stored-in-body.
7. Ibid.

Chapter 3: Your Birthday and the Protocol

1. Maggie Fox, "More Babies Die on Their First Day Than in 68 Other Countries, Report Shows," *NBC News*, April 30, 2013, https://www .nbcnews.com/healthmain/more-us-babies-die-their-first-day-68-other -countries-6C9700437.
2. Catharine Paddock, "Why Breastfeeding in the First Hour of Life Is Important," *Medical News Today*, August 1, 2007, https://www.medicalnewstoday.com /articles/78485#1.
3. Peeples, "Medicine's Secret Ingredient."
4. Pietro Cortelli, "Chronomedicine: A Necessary Concept to Manage Human Diseases," *Sleep Medicine Reviews* 21 (June 2015): 1–2, doi: 10.1016/j .smrv.2015.01.005.
5. Jonathan Shaw, "Raw and Red Hot," *Harvard Magazine*, May–June 2019, https:// harvardmagazine.com/2019/05/inflammation-disease-diet.
6. Oscar Castanon-Cervantes et al., "Disregulation of Inflammatory Response by Chronic Circadian Disruption," *Journal of Immunology* 185, no. 10 (November 2010): 5796–805, doi: 10.4049/jimmunol.1001026.
7. "The Dubious Practice of Detox," *Harvard Women's Health Watch*, May 2008, https://www.health.harvard.edu/staying-healthy/the-dubious-practice-of-detox.
8. David Pride, "Viruses Can Help Us as Well as Harm Us," *Scientific American*,

December 1, 2020, https://www.scientificamerican.com/article/viruses-can-help
-us-as-well-as-harm-us/.

9. Simin Sharifi et al., "Stem Cell Therapy: Curcumin Does the Trick," *Phytotherapy Research* 33, no. 11 (November 2019): 2927–37, https://doi.org/10.1002/ptr.6482.

Chapter 4: Making the Protocol Work for You

1. "Healthy Food for Babies," Generics Pharmacy, accessed April 7, 2021, https://tgp .com.ph/blog/healthy-food-babies/.

2. Kevin B. Comerford et al., "The Role of Avocados in Complementary and Transitional Feeding," *Nutrients* 8, no 5 (May 2016): 316, doi: 10.3390/nu8050316.

3. Ibid.

4. Anna Nekrich, "The Powerful Health Benefits of Citrus Fruits," *Whole U*, University of Washington, August 31, 2020, https://thewholeu .uw.edu/2020/08/31/citrus/.

5. David Fast et al., "Flavanones Common to Citrus Fruits Activate the Interferon-Stimulated Response Element by Stimulating Expression of IRF7," *Journal of Food Bioactives* 8 (December 2019): 58–65, DOI: 10.31665/JFB.2019.8207.

6. Jung-Kook Song and Jong-Myon Bae, "Citrus Fruit Intake and Breast Cancer Risk: A Quantitative Systematic Review," *Journal of Breast Cancer* 16, no. 1 (March 2013): 72–76, doi: 10.4048/jbc.2013.16.1.72.

7. "What Foods Cleanse Your Liver?" Fisher Titus, June 12, 2018, https://www .fishertitus.org/health/what-foods-cleanse-your-liver.

8. Eduardo Madrigal-Santillan, "Review of Natural Products with Hepatoprotective Benefits," *World Journal of Gastroenterology* 20, no, 40 (October 2014): 14787–804, doi: 10.3748/wjg.v20.i40.14787.

9. "Leafy Greens: Inflammation Fighters!" Oldways Nutrition Exchange, accessed April 7, 2021, https://oldwayspt.org/system/files/atoms/files/FoodMed _LeafyGreens.pdf.

10. "Anti-Inflammatory Diet Tip: Leafy Greens," Sharecare, accessed April 7, 2021, https://www.sharecare.com/health/inflammation/article/tip-4-greens.

11. "Chlorophyll and Chlorophyllin," Oregon State University, accessed April 7, 2021, https://lpi.oregonstate.edu/mic/dietary-factors/phytochemicals/chlorophyll -chlorophyllin.

12. Zhi Yu et al., "Associations Between Nut Consumption and Inflammatory Biomarkers," *American Journal of Clinical Nutrition* 104, no. 3 (September 2016): 722–28, doi: 10.3945/ajcn.116.134205.

13. Seunghyeon Kim et al., "Uncovering the Nutritional Landscape of Food," *PLoS ONE* 10, no. 4 (March 2013): https://doi.org/10.1371/journal.pone.0118697.

14. Jillian Levy, "Aflatoxin: How to Avoid This Common Food Carcinogen," Dr. Axe, May 2, 2016, https://draxe.com/nutrition/aflatoxin/.

15. Jennifer Warner, "Antioxidant Riches Found in Unexpected Foods," WebMD, June 17, 2004, https://www.webmd.com/food-recipes/news/20040617/antioxidants -found-unexpected-foods#1.

16. "Black Beans High in Antioxidant Ratings," NutraIngredients.com, December 10,

2003, https://www.nutraingredients.com/Article/2003/12/10/Black-beans-high
-in-antioxidant-ratings.

17. Jacqueline K. Innes and Philip C. Calder, "Omega-6 Fatty Acids and
    Inflammation," *Prostaglandins, Leukotrienes and Essential Fatty Acids* 132 (May
    2018): 41–48, https://doi.org/10.1016/j.plefa.2018.03.004.

18. Jerzy Z. Nowak, "Oxidative Stress, Polyunsaturated Fatty Acids-Derived
    Oxidation Products and Bisretinoids as Potential Inducers of CNS Diseases: Focus
    on Age-Related Macular Degeneration," *Pharmacological Reports* 65, no. 2 (2013):
    288–304, doi: 10.1016/s1734-1140(13)71005-3.

19. Tim Cutliffe, "Sunflower Oil Consumption Linked to Liver Damage in Rats,"
    Nutraingredients.com, February 7, 2018, https://www.nutraingredients.com
    /Article/2018/02/07/Sunflower-oil-consumption-linked-to-liver-damage-in
    -rats.

20. Josh Axe, "20 Coconut Oil Benefits for Your Brain, Heart, Joints + More!" Dr.
    Axe, April 24, 2019, https://draxe.com/nutrition/coconut-oil-benefits/#Health
    _Benefits.

21. Z. A. Zakaria et al., "Hepatoprotective Activity of Dried- and Fermented-
    Processed Virgin Coconut Oil," *Evidence-Based Complementary and Alternative
    Medicine* (2011), doi: 10.1155/2011/142739.

22. Nuray Z. Unlu et al., "Carotenoid Absorption from Salad and Salsa by Humans Is
    Enhanced by the Addition of Avocado or Avocado Oil," *Journal of Nutrition*, 135,
    no. 3 (March 2005): 431–36, doi: 10.1093/jn/135.3.431.

23. M. A. Cake et al., "Modification of Articular Cartilage and Subchondral Bone
    Pathology in an Ovine Meniscectomy Model of Osteoarthritis by Avocado and
    Soya Unsaponifiables," *Osteoarthritis Cartilage* 8, no. 6 (November 2000): 404–11,
    doi: 10.1053/joca.1999.0315.

24. Lana Barhum, "Can People with Type 2 Diabetes Eat Honey?" *Medical News
    Today*, December 22, 2020, https://www.medicalnewstoday.com/articles/317662#
    _noHeaderPrefixedContent.

25. K. U. Leuven, "Researchers Unravel How Stevia Controls Blood Sugar
    Levels," *ScienceDaily*, April 11, 2017, https://www.sciencedaily.com
    /releases/2017/04/170411104441.htm.

26. S. A. Kedik, E. I. Yartsev, and I. E. Stanishevskaya, "Antiviral Activity of Dried
    Extract of *Stevia*," *Pharmaceutical Chemistry Journal* 43, no. 4 (August 2009):198–
    99, doi: 10.1007/s11094-009-0270-7.

27. P. A. S. Theophilus et al., "Effectiveness of *Stevia rebaudiana* Whole Leaf Extract
    Against the Various Morphological Forms of *Borrelia burgdorferi* in Vitro,"
    European Journal of Microbiology & Immunology 5, no. 4 (December 2015): 268–80,
    doi:10.1556/1886.2015.00031.

28. "Hidden in Plain Sight," Sugar Science, University of California San Francisco,
    accessed April 7, 2021, https://sugarscience.ucsf.edu/hidden-in-plain-sight/#
    .X7QnZNNKhmA.

29. Jeffrey Norris, "Sugar Is a Poison, Says USCF Obesity Expert," University of San
    Francisco, June 25, 2009, https://www.ucsf.edu/news/2009/06/8187/obesity-and
    -metabolic-syndrome-driven-fructose-sugar-diet.

30. "Surprising Things That Can Damage Your Liver," WebMD, accessed April 7, 2021, https://www.webmd.com/hepatitis/ss/slideshow-surprising-liver-damage.

31. James J. DiNicolantonio and Amy Berger, "Added Sugars Drive Nutrient and Energy Deficit in Obesity: A New Paradigm," *Open Heart* 3, no. 2 (August 2016), doi:10.1136/openhrt-2016-000469.

32. Anne Alexander, "How Sugar Keeps Your Body from Detoxifying Naturally," *Prevention*, April 13, 2015, https://www.prevention.com/health/a20452897/how-sugar-damages-your-liver/.

33. Lisa Rapaport, "Eating Lots of Meat Tied to Higher Risk of Liver Disease," Reuters, February 12, 2019, https://www.reuters.com/article/us-health-liver-diet/eating-lots-of-meat-tied-to-higher-risk-of-liver-disease-idUSKCN1Q12T8.

34. Carl Engelking, "Red Meat Increases Cancer Risk Because of Toxic Immune Response," *Discover*, January 2, 2015, https://www.discovermagazine.com/health/red-meat-increases-cancer-risk-because-of-toxic-immune-response.

35. "Lactose Intolerance," Medline Plus, accessed April 8, 2021, https://medlineplus.gov/genetics/condition/lactose-intolerance/#frequency.

36. Rachel Link, "Goat Milk Benefits Are Superior to Cow Milk," Dr. Axe, November 22, 2018, https://draxe.com/nutrition/goat-milk/#Goat_Milk_vs_Cow_Milk_vs_Sheep_Milk.

37. Ibid.

38. Thomas Cook, "Benefits of Goat Milk vs. Cow Milk," Mt. Capra, August 20, 2010, https://mtcapra.com/benefits-of-goat-milk-vs-cow-milk.

39. Ethan Boldt, "What Are Nightshade Vegetables? How to Find Out If You're Sensitive to Them," Dr. Axe, April 25, 2018, https://draxe.com/nutrition/nightshade-vegetables/.

40. Roberto A. Ferdman, "How Corn Made Its Way into Just About Everything We Eat," *Washington Post*, July 14, 2015, https://www.washingtonpost.com/news/wonk/wp/2015/07/14/how-corn-made-its-way-into-just-about-everything-we-eat/.

41. Zawn Villines, "Is Corn Healthful?" *Medical News Today*, January 16, 2019, https://www.medicalnewstoday.com/articles/324199#health-concerns.

42. Louise Elizabeth Maher-Johnson and Ayana Elizabeth Johnson, "Broccoli Is Dying. Corn Is Toxic. Long Live Microbiomes!" *Scientific American*, August 20, 2019, https://blogs.scientificamerican.com/observations/broccoli-is-dying-corn-is-toxic-long-live-microbiomes/.

43. Amanda Kimber-Evans, "Genetically Modified Corn: Safe or Toxic?" *Mother Earth News*, https://www.motherearthnews.com/nature-and-environment/environmental-policy/genetically-modified-corn-zmaz10amzraw.

44. Ciddi Veeresham, "Natural Products Derived from Plants as a Source of Drugs," *Journal of Advanced Pharmaceutical Technology & Research* 3, no. 4 (October–December 2012): 200–201, doi: 10.4103/2231-4040.104709.

45. Judy McBride, "B$_{12}$ Deficiency May Be More Widespread Than Thought," US Department of Agriculture Agricultural Research Service, August 2, 2020, https://www.ars.usda.gov/news-events/news/research-news/2000/b12-deficiency-may-be-more-widespread-than-thought/.

46. Kris Gunnars, "10 Proven Health Benefits of Turmeric and Curcumin," Healthline, July 13, 2018, https://www.healthline.com/nutrition/top-10-evidence-based -health-benefits-of-turmeric.

47. Vilai Kuptniratsaikul et al., "Efficacy and Safety of Curcuma Domestic Extracts Compared with Ibuprofen in Patients with Knee Osteoarthritis: A Multicenter Study," *Clinical Interventions in Aging* 20, no. 9 (March 2014): 451–58, doi: 10.2147/CIA.S58535.

48. Nita Chainani-Wu, "Safety and Anti-Inflammatory Activity of Curcumin: A Component of Turmeric (*Curcuma longo*)," *Journal of Alternative and Complementary Medicine* 9, no. 1 (February 2003): 161–68.

49. Ying Xu et al., "Curcumin Reverses the Effects of Chronic Stress on Behavior, the HPA Axis, BDNF Expression and Phosphorylation of CREB," *Brain Research* 1122, no 1 (November 2006): 56–66, https://doi.org/10.1016/j .brainres.2006.09.009.

50. Wanwarang Wongcharoen and Arintaya Phrommintikul, "The Protective Role of Curcumin in Cardiovascular Diseases," *International Journal of Cardiology* 133, no. 2 (April 2009): 145–51, doi: 10.1016/j.ijcard.2009.01.073.

51. Preetha Anand et al., "Curcumin and Cancer: An 'Old-Age' Disease with an 'Age-Old' Solution," *Cancer Letters* 267, no. 1 (August 2008): 133–63, doi: 10.1016/j .canlet.2008.03.025.

52. Ji H. Kim et al., "Turmeric (*Curcuma longa*) Inhibits Inflammatory Nuclear Factor (NF)-κB and NF-κB-Regulated Gene Products and Induces Death Receptors Leading to Suppressed Proliferation, Induced Chemosensitization, and Suppressed Osteoclastogenesis." *Molecular Nutrition & Food Research* 56, no. 3 (March 2012): 454–65. doi:10.1002/mnfr.201100270.

53. Susan J. Hewlings and Douglas S. Kalman, "Curcumin: A Review of Its Effects on Human Health," *Foods* 6, no. 10 (October 2017): 92, doi: 10.3390 /foods6100092.

54. Lauren Bedosky, "Turmeric vs. Curcumin: Which Supplement Should You Take?" Everyday Health, March 4, 2020, https://www.everydayhealth.com/diet-nutrition /turmeric-vs-curcumin-which-supplement-should-you-take/.

55. Appian Subramoniam et al., "Chlorophyll Revisited: Anti-Inflammatory Activities of Chlorophyll A and Inhibition of Expression of TNF-α Gene by the Same," *Inflammation* 35, no. 3 (June 2012): 959–66, doi:10.1007/s10753-011-9399-0.

56. Bitna Yi et al., "Inhibition by Wheat Sprout (*Triticum aestivum*) Juice of Bisphenol A-Induced Oxidative Stress in Young Women," *Mutation Research* 724, no. 1–2 (September 2011): 64–68, doi: 10.1016/j.mrgentox.2011.06.007.

57. Noorjahan Banu Alitheen, "Cytotoxic Effects of Commercial Wheatgrass and Fiber Towards Human Acute Promyelocytic Leukemia Cells," *Pakistan Journal of Pharmaceutical Services* 24, no. 3 (July 2011): 243–50.

58. "The Gut-Brain Connection," *Healthbeat*, March 2012, https://www.health .harvard.edu/diseases-and-conditions/the-gut-brain-connection.

59. Lauren Bedosky, "The Absolute Best Time to Take Your Supplements," Parsley Health, December 22, 2020, https://www.parsleyhealth.com/blog/best-time-to -take-probiotics/.

60. Hiroshi Kunugi and Amira Mohammed Ali, "Royal Jelly and Its Components Promote Healthy Aging and Longevity: From Animal Models to Humans," *International Journal of Molecular Science* 20, no. 19 (October 2019): 4662, doi: 10.3390/ijms20194662.

61. Meng-Meng You et al., "Royal Jelly Attenuates LPS-Induced Inflammation in BV-2 Microglial Cells through Modulating NF-κB and p38/JNK Signaling Pathways," *Mediators of Inflammation* (April 2018), doi:10.1155/2018/7834381.

62. Hye Min Park et al., "Royal Jelly Increases Collagen Production in Rat Skin After Ovariectomy," *Journal of Medicinal and Food* 15, no. 6 (June 2012): 568–75, doi: 10.1089/jmf.2011.1888.

63. Juyoung Kim et al., "Royal Jelly Enhances Migration of Human Dermal Fibroblasts and Alters the Level of Cholesterol and Sphinganine in an Invitro Wound Healing Model," *Nutrition Research and Practice* 4, no. 5 (October 2010): 362–68, doi: 10.4162/nrp.2010.4.5.362.

64. "Melissa Officinalis," ScienceDirect, accessed April 8, 2021, https://www .sciencedirect.com/topics/medicine-and-dentistry/melissa-officinalis.

65. Amina Bounihi et al., '*In Vivo* Potential Anti-Inflammatory Activity of *Melissa officinalis* L. Essential Oil," *Advances in Pharmacological Science* (2013): 101759, doi: 10.1155/2013/101759.

66. Christa Sinadinos, "Herbal Therapeutic Treatments for Hypothyroidism," American Herbalists Guide, https://www.americanherbalistsguild.com/sites /default/files/sinadinos_christa_-_herbal_support_for_hypothyroidism.pdf.

67. Andrew Scholey et al., "Anti-Stress Effects of Lemon Balm-Containing Foods," *Nutrients* 6, no. 11 (October 2014): 4805–21, https://doi.org/10.3390/nu6114805.

68. Elaine Perry and Melanie-Jayne R. Howes, "Medicinal Plants and Dementia Therapy: Herbal Hopes for Brain Aging?" *CNS Neuroscience & Therapeutics* 17, no. 6 (December 2011): 683–98, doi: 10.1111/j.1755-5949.2010.00202.x.

69. "Milk Thistle," Stanford Children's Health, accessed April 8, 2021, https://www .stanfordchildrens.org/en/topic/default?id=milk-thistle-19-MilkThistle.

70. F. Galhardi et al., "Effect of Silymarin on Biochemical Parameters of Oxidative Stress in Aged and Young Rat Brain," *Food and Chemical Toxicology* 47, no. 10 (October 2009): 2655–60, doi: 10.1016/j.fct.2009.07.030.

71. Christos E. Kazazis, "The Therapeutic Potential of Milk Thistle in Diabetes," *Review of Diabetic Studies* 11, no. 2 (Summer 2014): 167–74, doi: 10.1900/ RDS.2014.11.167.

72. Joaquim Bosch-Barrera and Javier A. Menendez, "Silibinin and STAT3: A Natural Way of Targeting Transcription Factors for Cancer Therapy," *Cancer Treatment Reviews* 41, no 6. (June 2015): 540–46, doi: 10.1016/j.ctrv.2015.04.008.

73. "Milk Thistle."

74. Dirleise Colle et al., "Antioxidant Properties of *Taraxacum officinale* Leaf Extract Are Involved in the Protective Effect Against Hepatoxicity Induced by Acetaminophen in Mice," *Journal of Medicinal Food* 15, no 6 (June 2012): 549–56, doi:10.1089/jmf.2011.0282.

75. Yoon-Jeoung Koh et al., "Anti-Inflammatory Effect of *Taraxacum officinale* Leaves on Lipopolysaccharide-Induced Inflammatory Responses in RAW 264.7

Cells," *Journal of Medicinal Food* 13, no. 4 (August 2010): 870–78, doi:10.1089/jmf.2009.1249.

76. Yuan-Yuan Jia et al., "*Taraxacum mongolicum* Extract Exhibits a Protective Effect on Hepatocytes and an Antiviral Effect Against Hepatitis B Virus in Animal and Human Cells," *Molecular Medicine Reports* 9, no. 4 (April 2014): 1381–87, doi:10.3892/mmr.2014.1925.

77. O. Kenny et al., "Characterization of Antimicrobial Extracts from Dandelion Root (*Taraxacum officinale*) Using LC-SPE-NMR," *Phytotherapy Research* 29, no. 4 (April 2015): 526–32, doi: 10.1002/ptr.5276.

78. John Villarreal et al., "A Retrospective Review of the Prehospital Use of Activated Charcoal," *American Journal of Emergency Medicine* 33, no. 1 (January 2015): 56–59, doi: 10.1016/j.ajem.2014.10.019.

79. David N. Juurlink, "Activated Charcoal for Acute Overdose: A Reappraisal," *British Journal of Clinical Pharmacology* 81, no. 3 (March 2016): 482–87, doi: 10.1111/bcp.12793.

80. "Vitamin B$_{12}$," National Institutes of Health Office of Dietary Supplements, accessed April 9, 2021, https://ods.od.nih.gov/factsheets/VitaminB12-HealthProfessional/.

81. Abdul Jabbar et al., "Vitamin B$_{12}$ Deficiency Common in Primary Hypothyroidism," *Journal of the Pakistan Medical Association* 58, no. 5 (May 2008): 258–61, https://pubmed.ncbi.nlm.nih.gov/18655403/.

82. Jarrod Cooper, "Can MTHFR Affect Your Thyroid and Be a Root Cause of Hashimoto's Disease?" Advanced Functional Medicine, March 4, 2020, https://advancedfunctionalmedicine.com.au/mthfr-and-hashimotos-disease/.

83. Anna Dittfeld et al., "A Possible Link Between the Epstein-Barr Virus Infection and Autoimmune Thyroid Disorders," *Central European Journal of Immunology* 41, no. 3 (October 2016): 297–301, doi: 10.5114/ceji.2016.63130.

84. Luiz Querino Caldas et al., "Uncaria Tomentosa in the Treatment of the *Herpes labialis*: Randomized Double-Blind Trial," 2010, http://www.dst.uff.br/revista22-2-2010/1%20-%20Uncaria.pdf.

85. "Red Raspberry Leaf," ScienceDirect, accessed April 9, 2021, https://www.sciencedirect.com/topics/medicine-and-dentistry/red-raspberry-leaf.

86. Ayman A. A. Ewies, "Folic Acid Supplementation: The New Dawn for Post-Menopausal Women with Hot Flashes," *World Journal of Obstetrics and Gynecology* 2, no. 4 (November 2013): 87–93, doi: 10.5317.

87. Alec Coppen and Christina Bolander-Gouaille, "Treatment of Depression: Time to Consider Folic Acid and Vitamin B$_{12}$," *Journal of Psychopharmacology* 19, no. 1 (January 2005): 59–65, doi: 10.1177/0269881105048899.

88. Venthan J. Mailoo and Sanketh Rampes, "Lysine for *Herpes simplex* Prophylaxis: A Review of the Evidence," *Integrative Medicine: A Clinician's Journal* 16, no. 3 (June 2017): 42–46, https://www.ncbi.nlm.nih.gov/pmc/articles/PMC6419779/.

89. Thiago Caon et al, "Antimutagenic and Antiherpetic Activities of Different Preparations of *Uncaria tomentosa* (Cat's Claw)," *Food and Chemical Toxicology* 66 (April 2015): 30–35, doi: 10.1016/j.fct.2014.01.013.

90. Luiz Querino A. Caldez et al, "*Uncaria tomentosa* in the Treatment of the

Herpes labialas: Randomized Double-Blind Trial," *Brazilian Journal of Sexually Transmitted Diseases* 22, no. 2, (August 2010): 57–59, http://www.dst.uff.br/revista22-2-2010/1%20-%20Uncaria.pdf.

91. "Cat's Claw," Mount Sinai, accessed April 9, 2021, https://www.mountsinai.org/health-library/herb/cats-claw.

92. "Cat's Claw," Health Encyclopedia, University of Rochester Medical Center, accessed April 9, 2021, https://www.urmc.rochester.edu/encyclopedia/content.aspx?contenttypeid=19&contentid=CatsClaw.

Chapter 5: The Emotional Part of the Protocol

1. Maria C. Norton et al., "Family Member Deaths in Childhood Predict Systematic Inflammation in Late Life," *Biodemography and Social Biology* 63, no. 2 (2017) 104–15, doi: 10.1080/19485565.2017.1281099.

2. Eckelkamp, "Can Trauma Really Be Stored."

3. Ronald Peters, "The Connection Between Spontaneous Remission of Cancer and MindBody Medicine," *Cancer Strategies Journal* (summer 2013), https://www.healmindbody.com/wp-content/uploads/2013/12/Peters-article-Cancer-Strategies.pdf.

4. John Upledger, "Releasing Emotions Trapped in the Tissues," Massage Today, September 1, 2020, https://www.massagetoday.com/articles/13825/Releasing-Emotions-Trapped-in-the-Tissues.

5. Debbie Hampton, "How Your Thoughts Change Your Brain, Cells, and Genes," *HuffPost*, March 23, 2016, https://www.huffpost.com/entry/how-your-thoughts-change-your-brain-cells-and-genes_b_9516176.

6. "Guided Imagery," Breastcancer.org, accessed April 9, 2021, https://www.breastcancer.org/treatment/comp_med/types/imagery.

7. Jo Merchant, "Heal Yourself by Harnessing Your Mind," *Discover*, May 23, 2014, https://www.discovermagazine.com/health/heal-yourself-by-harnessing-your-mind.

8. "Study Reveals the Neural Mechanics of Self-Affirmation," University of Pennsylvania Annenberg School for Communication, November 20, 2105, https://www.asc.upenn.edu/news-events/news/study-reveals-neural-mechanics-self-affirmation.

9. Christopher N. Cascio et al., "Self-Affirmation Activates Brain Systems Associated with Self-Related Processing and Reward and Is Reinforced by Future Orientation," *Social Cognitive and Affective Neuroscience* 11, no. 4 (April 2016): 621–29, doi: 10.1093/scan/nsv136.

Chapter 6: Preparing for and Personalizing the Protocol

1. "Get in Touch with Your Circadian Rhythm," WebMD, February 21, 2020, https://www.webmd.com/sleep-disorders/find-circadian-rhythm.

2. "Epstein-Barr: Scientists Decode Secrets of a Very Common Virus that Can Cause Cancer," *ScienceDaily*, December 15, 2010, www.sciencedaily.com/releases/2010/12/101215121905.htm.

3. Jennifer Nardella, "Naturopathic Infection Management in Disease Prevention," Nardella Clinic, November 19, 2018, http://www.nardellaclinic.com/2018/11/19/naturopathic-infection-management-in-disease-prevention/.

4. Andrea Y. Arikawa et al., "Sixteen Weeks of Exercise Reduces C-Reactive Protein Levels in Young Women," *Medicine and Science in Sports and Exercise* 43, no 6. (June 2011): 1002–9, doi: 10.1249/MSS.0b013e3182059eda.

5. Adrian Meule, "The Psychology of Food Cravings: The Role of Food Deprivation," *Current Nutrition Reports* 9 (2020): 251–57, https://doi.org/10.1007/s13668-020-00326-0.

6. Tess Catlett, "Biotin for Hair Growth: Does It Work?" *Healthline*, April 5, 2021, https://www.healthline.com/health/biotin-hair-growth#research.

7. Cathy Wong, "The Health Benefits of GABA Supplements," VeryWell Health, June 26, 2020, https://www.verywellhealth.com/gaba-what-should-i-know-about-it-89053.

8. Sian Ferguson, "CBD for Insomnia: Benefits, Side Effects, and Treatment," Healthline, May 11, 2020, https://www.healthline.com/health/cbd-for-insomnia#research.

9. "Is It Bad to Wear Your Sunglasses All the Time?" All About Vision, accessed April 13, 2021, https://www.allaboutvision.com/sunglasses/faq/is-it-harmful-to-wear-sunglasses-all-the-time/.

10. Lois Zoppi, "Sex Hormones in Meat and Dairy," *News Medical*, accessed April 13, 2021, https://www.news-medical.net/health/Sex-Hormones-in-Meat-and-Dairy-Products.aspx.

11. "Exercise Is an All-Natural Treatment for Depression," *Harvard Health Letter*, July 2013, https://www.health.harvard.edu/mind-and-mood/exercise-is-an-all-natural-treatment-to-fight-depression.

12. John Briley, "The Xanax Workout," *Washington Post*, October 23, 2001, https://www.washingtonpost.com/archive/lifestyle/wellness/2001/10/23/the-xanax-workout/c399f0d4-70c0-462e-a7ec-75ccd8f66e55/.

13. Glenda Lindseth, Brian Helland, and Julie Caspers, "The Effects of Dietary Tryptophan on Affective Disorder," *Archives of Psychiatric Nursing* 29, no. 2 (April 2015): 102–7, doi: 10.1016/j.apnu.2014.11.008.

14. Naveed Saleh, "Don't Drink Coffee with These Vitamins," MDLinx, August 14, 2020, https://www.mdlinx.com/article/don-t-drink-coffee-with-these-vitamins/2OI25UJKhJQllHAjBlNNQU.

15. George A. Eby and Karen L. Eby, "Rapid Recovery from Major Depression Using Magnesium Treatment," *Medical Hypotheses* 67, no. 2 (2006) 362–70, doi: 10.1016/j.mehy.2006.01.047.

16. Sue Penckofer et al., "Vitamin D and Depression: Where Is All the Sunshine?" *Issues in Mental Health Nursing* 31, no. 6 (June 2010): 385–93, doi: 10.3109/01612840903437657.

17. "5-4-3-2-1 Coping Technique for Anxiety," Behavioral Health Partners blog, University of Rochester Medical Center, April 2018, https://www.urmc.rochester.edu/behavioral-health-partners/bhp-blog/april-2018/5-4-3-2-1-coping-technique-for-anxiety.aspx.

18. "Health Benefits of Taking Probiotics," Harvard Health Publishing, Harvard Medical School, September 2005, https://www.health.harvard.edu/vitamins-and -supplements/health-benefits-of-taking-probiotics.

19. Todd Cooperman, Q&A on Probiotics and Refrigeration, Consumerlab.com, June 3, 2012, https://www.consumerlab.com/answers/which-probiotics-require -refrigeration/probiotic-refrigeration/#:~:text=Answer%3A,and%20after%20 they%20are%20purchased.&text=Many%20probiotic%20bacteria%20are%20 naturally,nutrients%20and%20a%20proper%20environment.

20. Abby Olena, "Probiotics' Effects on the Microbiome Vary Widely," *Scientist*, September 6, 2018, https://www.the-scientist.com/news-opinion/probiotics -effects-on-the-microbiome-vary-widely-64760.

21. "8 Reasons to Drink Lemon Water in the Morning," EcoWatch, October 1, 2018, https://www.ecowatch.com/benefits-of-lemon-water-2608637935.html.

22. "Viruses That Can Lead to Cancer," American Cancer Society, accessed April 13, 2021, https://www.cancer.org/cancer/cancer-causes/infectious-agents/infections -that-can-lead-to-cancer/viruses.html.

23. "MTHFR Gene, Folic Acid, and Preventing Neural Tube Defects," Centers for Disease Control and Prevention, accessed April 13, 2021, https://www.cdc.gov /ncbddd/folicacid/mthfr-gene-and-folic-acid.html.

24. Lilin He and Yongxiang Shen, "MTHFR C677T Polymorphism and Breast, Ovarian Cancer Risk: A Meta-Analysis of 19,260 Patients and 26,364 Controls," *OncoTargets and Therapy* 10 (2017): 227–38, doi: 10.2147/OTT.S121472.

25. Elana-Alina Moacă et al., "A Comparative Study of *Melissa officinalis* Leaves and Stems Ethanolic Extracts in Terms of Antioxidant, Cytotoxic, and Antiproliferative Potential," *Evidence-Based Complementary and Alternative Medicine* (May 2018): 7860456, doi:10.1155/2018/7860456.

26. "Marijuana and Cancer," American Cancer Society, accessed April 13, 2021, https://www.cancer.org/treatment/treatments-and-side-effects/complementary -and-alternative-medicine/marijuana-and-cancer.html.

27. G. Velasco, C. Sanchez, and M. Guzman, "Anticancer Mechanisms of Cannabinoids," *Current Oncology* Suppl. 2 (March 2016): S23–S32, doi: 10.3747 /co.23.3080.

28. Jennifer Berry, "What are the Benefits of Chlorophyll?" *Medical News Today*, July 4, 2018, https://www.medicalnewstoday.com/articles/322361#benefits.

29. "Can Acupuncture Treat Cancer? An Interview with TCM Oncology Specialist Dr. Erlene Chiang," American College of Traditional Chinese Medicine, July 27, 2018, https://www.actcm.edu/blog/acupuncture/can-acupuncture-treat -cancer/.

30. J. Zhu et al., "Cryo-Thermal Therapy Elicits Potent Anti-Tumor Immunity by Inducing Extracellular Hsp70-Dependent MDSC Differentiation," *Scientific Reports* 6 (June 2016): 27136, https://doi.org/10.1038/srep27136.

31. "The Effects of Infrared Saunas on Cancer Cells," excerpt from "The Truth About Cancer," Island Hyperbaric Centre, May 17, 2019, https://centrehyperbare.com /the-effect-of-infrared-saunas-on-cancer-cells/.

32. Janis Kelly, "Got Magnesium? Those with Heart Disease Should," WebMD,

November 9, 2000, https://www.webmd.com/heart-disease/news/20001109/got
-magnesium-those-with-heart-disease-should#1.

33. Sinemyiz Atalay, Iwona Jarocka-Karpowicz, and Elzbieta Skrzydlewska, "Antioxidative and Anti-Inflammatory Properties of Cannabidiol," *Antioxidants* 9, no. 1 (January 2020): 21, doi: 10.3390/antiox9010021.

34. "Exercise Lowers Mortality Rate in Patients with Heart Disease," *CardioSmart News*, American College of Cardiology, September 30, 2017, https://www
.cardiosmart.org/news/2017/9/exercise-lowers-mortality-risk-in-patients-with
-heart-disease#:~:text=The%20more%20exercise%20the%20better,risk%20in%20
heart%20disease%20patients.

35. I. I. Pototskii and E. V. Zabolotskaia, "Role of Yeast-like *Candida* Fungi in the Development of Diabetes Mellitus Accompanied by Vasculitis," *Vrachebnoe delo* (July 1971): 48–50, https://pubmed.ncbi.nlm.nih.gov/5123023/.

36. Bridget Montgomery, "Diabetes and Gastrointestinal Issues," Diabetes Council, accessed April 13, 2021, https://www.thediabetescouncil.com/diabetes-and
-gastrointestinal-issues/.

37. Andrea M. White and Carol S. Johnson, "Vinegar Ingestion at Bedtime Moderates Waking Glucose Concentrations in Adults with Well-Controlled Type 2 Diabetes," *Diabetes Care* 30, no. 11 (November 2007): 2814–15, https://doi
.org/10.2337/dc07-1062.

38. Ibid.

39. Priyanga Ranasinghe et al., "Zinc and Diabetes Mellitus: Understanding Molecular Mechanisms and Clinical Implications," *DARU Journal of Pharmaceutical Sciences* 23, no. 1 (2015): 44, doi: 10.1186/s40199-015-0127-4.

40. "Top Foods High in Chromium," Nourish by WebMD, accessed April 13, 2021, https://www.webmd.com/diet/foods-high-in-chromium#1.

41. "The Importance of Exercise When You Have Diabetes," *Healthbeat*, October 2018, https://www.health.harvard.edu/staying-healthy/the-importance-of
-exercise-when-you-have-diabetes.

42. Meilu Lui et al., "Acupuncture and Related Techniques for Type 2 Diabetes Mellitus," *Medicine* 98, no. 2 (January 2019): e14509, doi: 10.1097/
MD.0000000000014059.

43. Renfang Mao et al., "Association Study Between Methylenetetrahydrofolate Reductase Gene Polymorphisms and Graves' Disease," *Cell Biochemistry and Function* 28, no 7. (Otcober 2010): 585–90, doi: 10.1002/cbf.1694.

44. Sarah Russo, "Molecular Mimicry: The Role of Cannabis in Healing Autoimmune Disease," Fundacion Canna, accessed April 13, 2021, https://www.fundacion
-canna.es/en/molecular-mimicry-role-cannabis-healing-autoimmune
-disease#:~:text=Cannabidiol%20also%20slows%20down%20T,cell%20
damage%20from%20autoimmune%20attacks.

45. Kassem Sharif et al., "Physical Activity and Autoimmune Diseases: Get Moving and Manage the Disease," *Autoimmunity Reviews* 17, no. 1 (January 2018): 53–72, doi: 10.1016/j.autrev.2017.11.010.

Chapter 7: Day One: New Beginning

1. Thomas C. Fung et al., "Intestinal Serotonin and Fluoxetine Exposure Modulate Bacterial Colonization in the Gut," *Nature Microbiology* 4, (September 2019): 2064–73, doi: 10.1038/s41564-019-0540-4.
2. Kristi Lee Schatz, "Your Brain on Meditation," *Noteworthy: The Journal Blog*, February 11, 2019, https://blog.usejournal.com/your-brain-on-meditation-344a63efba73.
3. Eino Havas et al., "Lymph Flow Dynamics in Exercising Human Skeletal Muscle as Detected by Scintigraphy," *Journal of Physiology* 504, no. 1 (1997): 233–39.
4. "The Truth about Dry Brushing and What It Does for You," Health Essentials, Cleveland Clinic, January 26, 2015, https://health.clevelandclinic.org/the-truth-about-dry-brushing-and-what-it-does-for-you/.
5. Heather Alexander, "Exercise and the Lymphatic System," MD Anderson Cancer Center, November 2019, https://www.mdanderson.org/publications/focused-on-health/exercise-and-the-lymphatic-system.h20-1592991.html.
6. Yoshinori Tanaka et al.," Daily Ingestion of Alkaline Electrolyzed Water Containing Hydrogen Influences Human Health, Including Gastrointestinal Systems," *Medical Gas Research* 8, no. 4 (October-December 2018): 160–66, doi: 10.4103/2045-9912.248267.

Chapter 9: Day Three: Restore

1. "Are You Acidic or Alkaline?" Rose Wellness Center for Integrative Medicine, January 24, 2021, https://www.rosewellness.com/are-you-acidic-or-alkaline/.
2. Joseph Pizzorno, "Acidosis: An Old Idea Validated by New Research," *Integrative Medicine* 14, no. 1 (February 2015): 8–12.
3. Julia Swain, "Hypothermia and Blood pH," *Journal of American Medical Association Archives of Internal Medicine* 148, no. 7 (1988): 1643–46, doi:10.1001/archinte.1988.00380070125030.
4. Willem van Eden, "Diet and Anti-Inflammatory Effects of Heat Shock Proteins," *Endocrine, Metabolic & Immune Disorders Drug Targets* 15, no. 1 (2015): 31–36, doi: 10.2174/1871530314666140922145333.
5. Karsten Kruger, Thomas Reichel, and Carsten Zeilinger, "Role of Heat Shock Proteins 7090 in Exercise Physiology and Exercise Immunology and Their Diagnostic Potential in Sports," *Journal of Applied Physiology* 126, no. 4 (April 2019): 916–27, https://doi.org/10.1152/japplphysiol.01052.2018.
6. Willem van Eden et al., "The Enigma of Heat Shock Proteins in Immune Tolerance," *Frontiers in Immunology* 8 (November 2017): 1599, doi: 10.3389/fimmu.2017.01599.
7. Ana Gotter, "Benefits of Cryotherapy," Healthline, March 2, 2020, https://www.healthline.com/health/cryotherapy-benefits#overview.
8. Richard Beever, "Far-Infrared Saunas for Treatment of Cardiovascular Risk Factors," *Canadian Family Physician* 55, no. 7 (July 2009): 691–96.
9. Sara Lindberg, "Are Infrared Saunas Safe?" Healthline, February 26, 2020, https://www.healthline.com/health/infrared-sauna-dangers#tips.

10. Kiera Nachman, "6 Ancient Remedies Thought to Keep pH Levels in Balance," MindBodyGreen, December 27, 2015, https://www.mindbodygreen.com/0 -23011/6-ancient-remedies-to-help-alkalize-your-body-mind.html.
11. Grant Tinsley, "7 Benefits of High-Intensity Interval Training (HIIT)," Healthline, June 2, 2017, https://www.healthline.com/nutrition/benefits-of -hiit#TOC_TITLE_HDR_9.

Chapter 10: Day Four: Rebuild

1. Rekha B. Kumar, "Is Sitting All Day Bad for You?" interview by Health Matters, New York–Presbyterian, accessed April 13, 2021, https://healthmatters.nyp.org /is-too-much-sitting-harming-your-body/.
2. Kristen Ciccolini, "If Your Gut Could Talk: 10 Things You Should Know," Healthline, September 18, 2017, https://www.healthline.com/health/digestive -health/things-your-gut-wants-you-to-know.
3. Dr. Alex Rinehart, "Regularity Matters: The Top-to-Bottom Guide to Supporting Gut Motility Naturally," accessed April 13, 2021, https://info.dralexrinehart.com /articles/regularity-guide-support-gut-motility-naturally.

Chapter 11: Day Five: Preparation

1. "What Does the Research Say about Reflexology?" Taking Care of Your Health & Wellbeing, University of Minnesota, accessed April 13, 2021, https://www .takingcharge.csh.umn.edu/explore-healing-practices/reflexology/what-does -research-say-about-refloxology.
2. Cathy Wong, "The Benefits of Lymphatic Massage," VeryWell Health, October 8, 2020, https://www.verywellhealth.com/the-benefits-of-lymphatic-massage-89857.
3. Giampietro L. Vairo et al., "Systematic Review of Efficacy for Manual Lymphatic Drainage Techniques in Sports Medicine and Rehabilitation: An Evidence-Based Practice Approach," *Journal of Manual & Manipulative Therapy* 17, no. 3 (2009): e80–e89, doi:10.1179/jmt.2009.17.3.80E.

Chapter 12: Day Six: Flush

1. "Top 5 Jobs Kidneys Do," National Kidney Foundation, accessed April 13, 2021, https://www.kidney.org/kidneydisease/top-5-jobs-kidneys-do.
2. Annie Price, "Epsom Salt: The Magnesium-Rich Detoxifying Pain Reliever," Dr. Axe, November 29, 2018, https://draxe.com/nutrition/epsom-salt/.
3. Jill Seladi-Schulman, "Are Essential Oils Useful for Hangovers? 3 Types to Try Out," Healthline, May 15, 2020, https://www.healthline.com/health/essential-oils -for-hangover#lavender.

Chapter 13: Day Seven: Rebirth

1. Judith Orloff, "The Health Benefits of Tears," *Psychology Today*, July 27, 2010, https://www.psychologytoday.com/us/blog/emotional-freedom/201007/the -health-benefits-tears.

2. Michelle Persad, "The Average Woman Puts 515 Synthetic Chemicals on Her Body Every Day Without Knowing," *HuffPost*, April 4, 2016, https://www.huffpost.com/entry/synthetic-chemicals-skincare_n_56d8ad09e4b0000de403d995.

3. Jeanne Lenzer, "Fatty Liver: Another Scary Reason to Lose Weight Today," AARP, March 18, 2021, https://www.aarp.org/health/conditions-treatments/info-2021/fatty-liver-disease.html.

4. "Embryologist Kim Tremblay Will Explore the Secrets of Liver Regeneration," News & Media Relations, University of Massachusetts Amherst, December 9, 2020, https://www.umass.edu/newsoffice/article/embryologist-kim-tremblay-will-explore#:~:text=%E2%80%9CUnlike%20any%20of%20our%20other,seven%20days%2C%E2%80%9D%20she%20says.&text=In%20the%20embryonic%20liver%20bud,cell%20types%20%E2%80%93%20hepatocytes%20and%20cholangiocytes.

5. "4 Things You Should Know about Colon Cleansing," Health Essentials, July 8, 2020, https://health.clevelandclinic.org/colon-cleansing-is-it-safe/#:~:text=Colon%20cleansing%2C%20also%20called%20colonic,lethargy%2C%20asthma%20and%20skin%20conditions.

6. MaryAnn De Pietro, "What Are the Health Benefits of Epsom Salt Foot Soaks?" Healthline, September 19, 2019, https://www.medicalnewstoday.com/articles/epsom-salt-foot-soak#how-to-do-it.

Chapter 14: Maintaining the Protocol

1. Meg Selig, "Why Diets Don't Work . . . and What Does," *Psychology Today*, October 21, 2010, https://www.psychologytoday.com/us/blog/changepower/201010/why-diets-dont-work-and-what-does.

INDEX

detox belly, 162, 173

detoxification. *See also* Cleanse;
    inflammation-detoxification cycle
  avoiding invasive procedures during, 175
  benefits of, 46–47
  birth process and, 37
  body growth and healing using, 24
  cheat meals and, 154
  chemotherapy and, 124
  chronic inflammation and, 44
  circaseptan rhythms and, 3–4
  citrus fruits for, 57, 58
  coconut and avocado cooking oil and, 59
  cow's dairy and, 62
  Day Five for preparing for, 42, 185
  Day One recovery from, 28, 108–9, 151,
    171
  Day Seven and, 32, 40, 44, 64, 69–70,
    161
  Day Six and, 40, 44, 64, 69–70
  detox belly in, 162, 173
  dietary sugar and, 61
  EBV and CMV infection and, 103
  exercise and, 42, 177
  food choice and nutrition in, 41, 55,
    170, 173, 179, 184
  increasing body's ability to, 45–46
  inflammation reduction using, 20
  liver and, 31, 45, 55, 59, 61, 142, 152,
    161, 162, 171–72, 179
  physiological processes in Stage Two
    and, 30–31
  Protocol's benefits for, 38
  red meat and, 61
  seven-day cycles of, 4, 14–15, 23
  stretching and, 177
  supplement usage interfering with, 41
  supplements for boosting, 55, 63, 64,
    69–70, 94, 184, 185

diabetes
  approaches to helping, 105
  coronavirus pandemic and, 39
  inflammation and, 24, 44, 181
  Protocol's benefits for, 38
  supplements for, 105

diagnostic testing, scheduling, 111–12, 123,
  165, 175

dialysis, scheduling, 155

diet and food choices
  cancer management and, 104
  cheat meals and, 154, 184
  circaseptan rhythms and, 41, 52, 55, 97
  Cleanse and, 56
  C-reactive protein (CRP) levels and, 96
  Day Five, 160
  Day Four, 148, 150
  Day One, 111, 117
  Day Seven, 179–80
  Day Six, 169–70
  Day Three, 138–39
  Day Two, 123, 127
  detoxification and, 41, 55, 170, 173, 179,
    184
  food sensitivities and, 147–48
  inflammation caused by, 56, 168
  inflammation reduction using, 44, 48, 55,
    98, 158
  lab-engineered chemicals and hormones
    in, 62, 172
  maintaining, 183–84
  minimizing proinflammatory foods in,
    55, 56, 60–63, 184, 185
  nonalcoholic fatty liver disease (NAFLD)
    and, 173
  patience in adopting new approach to, 187
  prioritizing healthy foods in, 57–60, 93,
    184, 185
  proinflammatory foods in, 56, 60, 182,
    184, 186
  Protocol recommendations for, 38, 44, 48,
    53, 93, 185
  role of, in the Protocol, 41, 55–56, 97,
    183–84
  seven-day cycle for timing of, 26
  sleep quality and, 99
  supplements used with, 55, 64, 184. *See
    also* supplements
  syncing with circaseptan rhythms, 64, 92,
    97, 181
  three *d* Protocol approach using, 182, 186
  toxins in, 17
  weight loss and, 97

digestive problems
  approaches to helping, 103
  chronic inflammation and, 24
  circadian-rhythm interruptions and, 2

inflammation (*cont.*)
  minimizing unhealthy foods in, 55, 56, 60–63, 184, 185
  proinflammatory foods promoting, 56, 60, 182, 184, 186
  seven-day cycles of, 14–15, 22, 24–25
  sleep-wake cycle interruptions and, 2
inflammation-detoxification cycle
  birth process and beginning of, 37
  body growth and healing using, 24
  importance of knowing your cycle in, 4, 25
  personal story about experience of, 51–52
  personalizing the Protocol for, 53–54
  Protocol's benefits for, 53
  seven-day cycles in, 4, 22–23, 25, 35
  syncing daily activities with, 26–27, 74
  two stages in, 27
  using to your advantage, 26–27
inflammation reduction
  benefits of, 46–47
  detoxification and, 44
  diet and, 44, 48, 55, 98, 158
  lymphatic massage and, 156
  Protocol for, 43–45
  supplements for, 41, 135, 173
infrared saunas, 104, 134–35, 136
insulin resistance, 105, 173
intravenous treatments, 111
invasive procedures, scheduling, 40, 123, 165, 175, 183

journaling, 32, 79–80, 84, 94, 110
  Day Seven with, 174
  recording and celebrating your progress with, 185

kickboxing classes, 146–47
kidney disease
  acidic blood and, 130
  dialysis and, 155
  heat therapy risk in, 135
kidneys
  birth process and, 37
  Cleanse and, 24, 45, 55, 56, 172, 184
  Day Five and, 30, 151, 152
  Day One recovery and, 108
  Day Six and, 30, 31, 161–62, 163, 165, 168, 172

detoxification process and, 45, 55, 161
  emotional trauma affecting, 86
  Epsom salt baths and, 31
  exercise and, 167
  food choices and nutrition and, 55
  hydration and, 31, 164, 177
  proinflammatory foods and, 56
  Protocol's benefits for, 46
  reflexology for, 156
  supplements for, 169, 184
  toxin flushing by, 45, 172
  worry and anxiety and, 81, 86
kidney stones, 167–68, 169
knees, and feeling unable or having an inability to move forward, 83, 88

lemon balm
  days used, 104, 116, 126, 132, 149
  description of, 68–69
lentils, 59
Lipton, Bruce, 20
listening to your body, 33, 47, 91, 95, 174–75, 189
literature, number seven in, 14
liver
  acupuncture and, 104
  anger and, 81, 86
  birth process and, 37
  citrus fruits and, 58
  Cleanse and, 24, 30, 31, 45, 55, 56, 172, 184
  colonics and, 176
  cooking oils and, 59
  dandelion root for, 69, 169
  Day Five and, 30, 151, 152, 155
  Day Four rebuilding and, 29, 129, 131, 142
  Day One recovery and, 28, 108–9
  Day Seven and, 30, 162, 172, 173–74, 176
  Day Six and, 30, 161
  Day Two and, 120
  detox belly and, 162, 173
  detoxification and, 31, 45, 55, 59, 61, 142, 152, 161, 162, 171–72, 179
  dietary sugar and, 61
  emotional trauma affecting, 86, 174
  exercise and, 137
  food choice and, 55, 56, 150, 170, 179–80
  foot soak release of toxins and, 176
  genetically modified (GM) foods and, 63

Miller, George, 11
mood
    alcohol and caffeine intake and, 102
    being in sync with circadian rhythms
        to improve, 93
    checking iron, ferritin, and vitamin B_{12}
        levels in, 102
    impact of circadian-rhythm interruptions
        to, 1
    impact of circaseptan rhythms on, 19
    lunar cycles affecting, 8
    microbiome's influence on, 8, 44, 64, 67
    probiotics and, 64, 67–68
    Protocol's improvement to, 43
    serotonin's influence on, 72, 102, 108
    sugar's impact on, 61
    supplements for help with, 102
    vitamin B_{12} and, 71–72, 102
    woman's menstrual cycles and, 9
moon
    circaseptan rhythms and phases of, 8, 13
    influence of cycles of, 8
    seven-day week cycle based on phases
        of, 7–8

nails
    approaches to helping problems
        in, 98
    Day 4 rebuilding for, 29, 131, 142
    manicures and pedicures for, 146
    Protocol's benefits for, 43, 47, 53
    thyroid problems and, 98
National Institutes of Health (NIH), 3
nature, number seven in, 13
naturopathic medicine, 1, 39
neurotrophic factor, 66
nightshade vegetables, 62–63
nonalcoholic fatty liver disease
        (NAFLD), 173
nutrition. See diet and food choices
nuts, 58–59

oil pulling, 135
oils, in cooking, 59–60
olive oil, 60
organ transplantation, seven-day cycle
        in, 10
orthopedic surgery, scheduling, 145

osteopath visits, 144–45
ovarian cancer, 78, 104

pain, chronic
    approaches to helping, 100–101
    cryotherapy for, 134
pancreas
    emotional trauma affecting, 86
    injury, illness, or conditions affecting, 81
pedicures, 146
perimenopause
    approaches to helping, 101
    supplements for, 71, 94, 101, 116, 127,
        138, 149, 160
personalizing the Protocol, 40, 53–54, 95–106
Pilates, 146
power lifting, 146
prediabetes
    approaches to helping, 105
    supplements for, 105
premature aging
    chronic inflammation and, 24
    circadian-rhythm interruptions and, 2
    Protocol's benefits for, 38
    royal jelly for, 68
probiotics, 64
    days used, 64, 116, 126, 137, 149, 159
    description of, 67–68
    stomach problems and, 103
progesterone, seven-day cycles in
        menstruation with, 9, 11
Protocol
    beauty benefits of, 47
    benefits of, 42–43
    creation of, 38–40
    daily snapshot of, 27–32
    Day Five in, 151–60
    Day Four in, 141–49
    Day One in, 107–17
    Day Seven in, 171–80
    Day Six in, 161–70
    Day Three in, 129–39
    Day Two in, 119–27
    detoxification ability increase in, 45–46
    emotional part of, 73–89
    exercise's role in, 41–42
    food and diet's role in, 41, 55–63, 97,
        183–84

shoulders, and feeling burdened or guarded, 88, 93, 100

skin
being in sync with circadian rhythms to improve, 93
Day 4 for scheduling treatments for, 146, 162
dry-brushing technique for, 112–13
Protocol's benefits for, 29, 30, 38, 43, 46, 47, 53, 131, 142
emotional trauma affecting, 87
injury, illness, or conditions affecting, 82

skin-care products, 98, 102, 163, 172–73

skin problems
antioxidants for repair in, 160
approaches to helping, 98
chronic inflammation and, 24
circadian-rhythm interruptions and, 2
colonics for, 176
Day Five for healing and regeneration in, 152, 156, 158
Day Four treatments for, 146
histamine levels in allergic reactions and, 120, 163
lymphatic massage for, 156
thyroid evaluation in, 98
thyroid supplements for help with, 98

sleep
being in sync with circadian rhythms to improve, 93
inflammation reduction using, 44
lunar cycles affecting, 8
need for sufficient amounts of, 32
Protocol's improvement to quality of, 43, 53, 179, 185
supplements for help with, 99
variables affecting, 99

sleeping pills, prescription, 99, 178, 179

sleep problems
alcohol and caffeine intake and, 102
approaches to helping, 99
chronic inflammation from, 24, 44
circadian-rhythm interruptions and, 44
circaseptan-rhythm interruptions and, 178
low energy or fatigue from, 99
weighted blankets for, 99
white noise for, 99

sleep-wake cycles
circadian rhythms and, 1, 7, 30, 44, 93
circaseptan rhythms and, 179
Day One after birth and, 107
eye photoreceptors for triggering, 100
impact of interruptions to, 2
tumor growth related to, 20–21

social activities, on Day Four, 144

spine
chiropractic adjustments to, 144–45
feeling unable or having an inability to stand up for yourself and, 88, 92
scheduling surgery for, 145

spiritual benefits of the Protocol, 49

Stage One, 28–30

Stage Two, 30–32

steam baths, 134

stevia, 60

stomach
aloe vera juice for settling, 103
anxiety or nervousness feelings in, 32
Day Four repair of, 142
Day One and, 28
feeling victimized or wounded or unable to acknowledge your power and, 81, 86
probiotics and, 68, 102
scheduling procedures for, 155
supplements for problems with, 103

strategic thinking, 132

stress
circadian-rhythm interruptions and, 2
day of birth and, 36–37
inflammation and, 24
sleep quality and, 99
sugar and, 60

stress management
body processes and, 26
Day One and, 28, 108, 111
Day Six and, 30, 31, 162–63, 164
inflammation reduction using, 44
Protocol's benefits for, 46, 48, 183
reflexology and, 156
sleep quality and, 99

stretching, 112, 177

sugar, dietary, 60–61

sugar substitutes, 60

ABOUT THE AUTHOR

DR. OLIVIA AUDREY is a board-certified doctor of natural medicine and an intuitive healer. Over the last decade, she has helped overhaul the health of dozens of A-list celebrities, professional athletes, and members of European royalty, along with the everyday patients whom she treats all over the world. Dr. Audrey grew up in the mountains of rural Maine, where she learned at a young age that all species are interconnected and that everything alive has the power to heal from within. She began her life's mission to empower and educate those in need of physical, emotional, or spiritual healing, and her work has won her the American Natural Medical Association's prestigious Outstanding Achievement award. When she isn't traveling the world sharing her gift, Dr. Audrey lives in coastal Maine with her three children and their dog, Bodhi. You can still find her exploring forests and forgotten woods, where she feels most at home among the trees.